Developing Reflective Practice

Developing Reflective Practice

A guide for medical students, doctors and teachers

Andrew Grant
Judy McKimm
Fiona Murphy

WILEY Blackwell

Contents

Acknowledgements

We would like to thank our students and many colleagues over the years in helping us to develop and shape the ideas set out in the book. In particular, we would like to acknowledgethe Swansea Medical School Graduate Entry Medicine and Leadership Masters' students who generously provided examples of reflective writing, the help given by Sam May in the authorship of Chapter 9 and the administrative support provided by Charly Cope. Finally, we would like to thank our partners (Alistair, Andy and Phil) and our families for their unfailing support for our writing endeavours.

About the Authors

Andrew Grant

Professor Andrew Grant is Dean of Medical Education at Swansea University Medical School. His PhD thesis (completed in 2005) was based on reflective learning in 3rd year medical students. He has gained experience with reflective learning in undergraduate medical education in a number of settings. As a practising GP, Andrew completes a portfolio for appraisal each year. This experience of having to keep a reflective portfolio has given him a great deal of insight into the practicalities of recording written reflections while working as a busy practitioner and educator. Andrew worked as a GP in North West London for ten years before moving into a full-time academic career in medical education.

Judy McKimm

Professor Judy McKimm is Director of Strategic Educational Development and Professor of Medical Education at Swansea University Medical School. From 2011–2014, she was Dean of Medical Education at Swansea and before that worked in New Zealand from 2007-2011, at the University of Auckland and as Pro-Dean, Health and Social Care, Unitec Institute of Technology. Judy initially trained as a nurse and has an academic background in social and health sciences, education and management. She was Director of Undergraduate Medicine at Imperial College London until 2004 and led the curriculum development and implementation of the new undergraduate medical programme. She has worked on over sixty international health workforce and education reform projects for DfID, AusAID, the World Bank and WHO in Central Asia, Portugal, Greece, Bosnia & Herzegovina, Macedonia, Australia and the Pacific. She writes and publishes widely on medical education, leadership and professional identity and runs health professions' leadership and education courses and workshops internationally.

Fiona Murphy

Professor Fiona Murphy is Professor of Clinical Nursing in the Department of Nursing and Midwifery at the University of Limerick. Before that she was an associate professor at Swansea University with extensive involvement in delivering programmes to healthcare practitioners at all levels. She has much experience in facilitating teaching and learning in reflective practice to healthcare professionals, in particular debriefing and analysis of critical incidents from clinical practice. Fiona trained as a nurse and public health nurse and has worked extensively in the United Kingdom, Ireland and the United States.

Part I

What is Reflection?

Perspectives on Reflection

If you are a student or doctor in training, it is very likely that you are reading this book because you have been told that reflection is now a required part of your learning, and that you are in some way expected to provide evidence of this reflective activity. The purpose of this book is to help you to use the time that you spend in this reflective activity in a way that is beneficial to you, to your learning, and to your skills as a learner and future practitioner. The book is also relevant (and we hope useful) for clinical and academic teachers who are interested in developing effective and meaningful reflective practices in their learners wherever they are in their stage of education or training, and for doctors at all stages of their career who have to engage in reflective activities for their continuing professional development. We set out the structure and give an overview of the content of each section and chapter of the book at the end of this chapter. Prior to that, each of us has set out a personal 'reflection on reflection' as part of setting the context for the book; these include some of the challenges for embedding reflective practice into programmes as well as some of the benefits.

Reflective Learning: Making a Difference – Andrew Grant

I was sufficiently interested in its possible applications to make reflective learning in undergraduate medical students the subject of my PhD. Studying the subject in depth taught me that reflection can enhance medical students' learning in a variety of ways.

My early work was largely focussed on reflection as a way of learning from experience. I used a number of techniques to help students to reflect on learning encounters and to identify the learning needs that were revealed. I have used templates based on the Kolb cycle (Kolb, 1984) as well as facilitated reflective learning groups (Grant, 2013) to support this form of learning. What I

Developing Reflective Practice: A guide for medical students, doctors and teachers, First Edition.
Andrew Grant, Judy McKimm and Fiona Murphy.
© 2017 John Wiley & Sons Ltd. Published 2017 by John Wiley & Sons Ltd.

discovered through my research in this area is that reflective learning helps learners to better integrate learning and to be more self-directed. When students are addressing learning needs that they have identified for themselves, their motivation is intrinsic. What reflection particularly offers medical students is a way of constantly modifying and adding to their body of knowledge, with the result that they are able not just to reproduce what they know but to apply it in future situations, which might be different from the context in which they first learned it. Medical students are faced with a wide, varied and interconnected body of knowledge that they have to master. Reflection offers them a potent tool, which allows them to take control of this process and to become much more aware of their body of knowledge at any one time: where its strengths lie and where the gaps are.

Further study of reflective learning showed me that the use of reflection as a way of managing what you know and what you need to know is just one facet of reflective learning, albeit an important one. As well as acquiring a body of knowledge that they can apply appropriately in multiple clinical contexts, medical students also have to undergo a degree of professional development. Through reflection on clinical encounters they can examine their own values and recognize the qualities that they will need to develop in order to think, speak, act and behave like doctors.

As reflection becomes a core learning activity for medical students and practising doctors at all stages of their careers, it forms an essential part of an increasing number of core learning activities. Of particular note is the way reflection is embedded in aspects of selection and forms part of professionalism. For example, as part of selection processes at undergraduate and for speciality training, applicants are typically asked to how they would approach a situation with a number of conflicting demands and explain and reflect on their choices. They may also be asked to reflect on significant events or ethical dilemmas they have faced, and discuss what they have learned from the process and how this would affect their future practice. Reflection is a key aspect of professionalism, but also in terms of how a lack of reflection and self-insight often underpins unprofessional behaviours. The General Medical Council (GMC) notes that 'the sort of misconduct, whether criminal or not, which indicates a lack of integrity on the part of the doctor, an unwillingness to practise ethically or responsibly or a serious lack of insight into obvious problems of poor practice will bring a doctor's registration into question' (GMC, 2014). Such behaviours (from students and practitioners) can lead to investigation by their medical school/university or the regulator. As part of the investigation or fitness to practise (FTP) process, they may be asked to give an account of the events and through reflection to demonstrate that they are able to show insight into their actions and the possible consequences. For example, the Doctors' Defence Service UK advises doctors who are required to attend a GMC FTP hearing to provide evidence of personal insight to support their case: 'a doctor should write out their reflections, giving careful thought to what they want to say, with a view to submitting their writings to the FTP panel. The exercise will also assist the doctor in presenting their case when they give oral evidence' (Doctors' Defence Service UK 2016). Whilst these examples are at the extreme end of the spectrum in terms of why reflection is important, they highlight its importance in maintaining professionalism throughout one's career, which is founded on self-insight, reflection and learning.

Start Early, Make it Routine – Judy McKimm

Working with doctors in training on postgraduate leadership programmes for over 10 years has caused me to think about the effectiveness of the training in purposeful reflection that occurs at undergraduate level and beyond. As with many masters' programmes, being able to reflect on and for action and think critically, and to link this meaningfully to practice, are key learning outcomes and 'transferable skills'. A few things come to mind when I think about how we embed reflection and critical thinking into the programme. The first is how little prepared (and often resistant) most of the students are to engage in formal reflective activities. Whilst they are more than happy to reflect on, in and for action through small group and whole class activities, when it comes to writing, especially writing for summative assessments, it becomes more challenging. Most students and doctors in training have not done purposeful reflection to any great extent, other than perhaps writing reflective accounts that do not get feedback or, whilst they have to be completed, are not marked summatively. So, one thought is that perhaps we need to educate teachers better on the different ways in which reflection can be embedded into a programme from the start, the ways in which reflection can be assessed (formally and informally, formatively and summatively) and how to overcome resistance in learners. Kurt Lewin says 'there's nothing as practical as a good theory' (Lewin, 1946), and I would paraphrase this to say 'there's nothing as practical as good reflection'. Fiona talks more below about some of the challenges, but my students would say (see some quotes in later chapters as well as this one) that the benefits far outweigh the challenges in terms of developing them as truly reflective practitioners.

So what do we do in the leadership programmes to help develop reflection as a routine learning and practice activity? First, we openly discuss the students' experiences of reflection (positive and negative) and set this in the context of the programme and its requirements. We know that 'assessment drives learning', and, because every written assignment has a reflective component included, this becomes a key motivation factor. We spend half a day with the students (out of eight contact days) on reflective practice and its importance for leadership development. This includes the theoretical background, some frameworks and models, the importance of triangulating experiences and observations with the leadership literature and what 'good' and 'poor' reflections look like, and, most importantly, students have time to practise and receive constructive feedback from tutors and peers on both oral and written reflective activities. Whilst we teach leadership 'theory', our main aim is something much broader than this, encapsulated in a written reflection from a student:

> I expected to gain knowledge, which would be directive to say, in this situation we do that, and in this situation we do this. But instead, it has given me a way of thinking, to tie any theory in with practice (K, C7).

Such a way of thinking has reflection at its heart. Throughout the course, we take a reflective approach to teaching, through questioning our own and others' practice; encouraging challenge and facilitating 'fierce conversations'; enabling students to learn more about themselves (their strengths and areas for development), and equipping students with different tools and techniques to 'think differently', critically and from different perspectives, such as de Bono's 'thinking hats', (de Bono, 1885) 'what if?' questions and 'empathy mapping'. A range of reflective and critical thinking assessments include: a 'significant event analysis', their 'leadership journey' reflective narrative, critical review of a leadership article, critique of effective and failing leadership, reflection on the way they managed their quality improvement project and critical reflection on themselves as 'change leaders'. The culmination of these activities is shown in the quote below from one of the students at the end of the first year of the clinical leadership programme:

> I think that the biggest development has been in deciphering what type of leader I am. I thought I knew, I thought I was aware of my strengths and weaknesses and had a good understanding of the traits and behaviours necessary to lead a team successfully. But what I have learnt is that I have become more self-aware, more able to appreciate the differences between the real and modelled worlds. I have developed the courage to challenge the status quo, to supress manipulating behaviour and to have the conviction to implement unpopular measures, I have learnt under what circumstances to exercise legitimate authority (A, C1).

If we can facilitate such deep reflections from our learners through embedding a curriculum philosophy, approach and activities that have reflection and critical thinking at its heart, then we will in turn develop the reflective practitioners of the future, who will have what Kouzes and Posner call 'the courage of the heart' (2009, p. 63) to challenge and improve healthcare.

Some Challenges for Reflective Practice – Fiona Murphy

Part of the purpose of this book is to articulate the positive contribution that reflective practice can make in both the initial preparation of practitioners and continuous professional development. Reflective practice is about not just teaching and learning, but fostering within individuals the skills of critical thinking and a constantly questioning approach, not just to their own practice but also to the context in which their practice occurs. A challenge for the exponents of reflective practice within a curriculum is how to ensure that reflective practice is not reduced to some meaningless tick-box exercise in which learners just go through the motions of reflecting and producing reflective material they think their teachers and assessors want to see. Sometimes, the process of reflecting is more important than the need to produce outcomes that satisfy some kind of external criterion. At its heart, reflective practice and the reflective practitioner both have the potential to be subversive, and it is this element of subversion that needs to be developed and channelled. Being able to be reflective enables the individual to appraise healthcare and healthcare practice in a 'critical' way and see it from different perspectives. This can enable challenges to dominant discourses within healthcare and offer alternatives. The challenges for healthcare educators are to ensure that these skills are developed in learners.

Another continuing challenge for reflective practice is 'show me the evidence that reflective practice works'. It is widely adopted within healthcare, but there is little empirical evidence that supports some of the claims made for it, apart from its widespread adoption. In an evidence-based healthcare system in which specific kinds of evidence are needed to demonstrate tangible outcomes, this is indeed seen as a deficiency. However, a counterargument to this is that not all forms of phenomenon readily lend themselves to being measured in such a reductionist way, so, despite this kind of evidence not being readily available, this does not indicate that it is not worth adopting. However, serious reservations as to the utility and efficacy of reflective practice exist, and these concerns need to be taken seriously and addressed.

Finally, in a fast-moving, globalized, social-media-dominated world, is reflecting in and on action still of relevance? The ability to access masses of information on a wide range of topics is a feature of contemporary society and healthcare. However, this information may be distorted and false, and hence there is even more of a need to pause and critically reflect on the nature of the information and its source. The skills of reflection – especially critical reflection – are therefore even more important in contemporary society and healthcare.

About the Book: Structure and Content Overview

The book is divided into four parts, each of which considers reflection and reflective activities from a different perspective:

Part 1   What is reflection?
Part 2   Learning reflection
Part 3   Facilitating reflection
Part 4   Developing as a reflective practitioner.

In Part 1, we describe and explore some of the theoretical underpinnings of reflection and reflective practice, and some frameworks and models that help guide and structure reflective activities. These are considered in relation to key educational, political and professional drivers that lie behind the current emphasis on ensuring doctors are reflective, mindful practitioners. Chapter 2 specifically considers reflection and reflective practice in their broadest sense, describing what these are (and what they are not). We look at the reasons why learners are asked to reflect and what they may expect to gain from reflective learning. We also explore differences between informal, everyday reflection and the more formal, structured learning activities in which many programmes require learners to engage, and describe some techniques for reflection. In Chapter 3, we build on this by taking a multidisciplinary, historical approach to exploring and explaining reflection for medical students, trainees and doctors, and explaining where reflective practice emerged from, in the context of major educational, philosophical and psychological perspectives including those of Dewey, Freire, Kolb, Vygotsky, Ausubel and Schön.

Part 2 is written specifically for learners and practitioners, providing guidance and ideas about how to embed reflection into day-to-day learning experiences and activities (reflecting in, on and for action), particularly in clinical practice. Chapter 4 considers a range of influential models and frameworks that have been, or are currently, used to structure, explain and develop reflection. The chapter describes these in terms of the contexts in which they may be helpful and considers their strengths and limitations, including the evidence base for each. In Chapter 5, we shift the focus to considering some practical activities that can help reflection in clinical practice, taking some of the theories and frameworks described in Chapters 3 and 4 and applying them to various contexts through case studies and examples. This chapter looks primarily at *reflection on action*, activities and models that can help practitioners capture and reflect on events that have already happened. Chapter 6 looks at writing as a reflective process in more depth. It looks at the range of activities, requirements and modalities involved in reflective writing, including informal, personal and formative reflection via journals, diaries, logs and e-portfolios and writing for summative assessments. In Chapter 7, we consider a range of face-to-face activities that occur in various learning and clinical settings which incorporate reflection. These might involve individual learners working on a one-to-one basis with a facilitator or teacher (such as appraisal, supervision, mentoring or coaching) or learners working in a small group of peers with a facilitator, for example in problem or case-based learning. Finally, in Chapter 8 we explore reflection as a way of developing and accessing knowledge about our own practice through research and critical inquiry. The chapter discusses reflection and knowledge generation, critical thinking and action research through practical examples and illustrations.

In Part 3 we move the focus to the perspective of the teacher, educator or trainer working as a facilitator of reflection in informal and formal settings, and with individuals or groups of learners. Chapter 9 looks at the curriculum or programme (be this at undergraduate, postgraduate or professional development level) and how reflection can be built into the curriculum through various approaches, activities and methods. The chapter also considers how the teacher might evaluate the impact or success of the curriculum initiatives. This chapter looks at specific learning and teaching methods that can be used to encourage, support and promote reflection and reflective practice. These include formal 'classroom' or clinically based activities, self-directed learning and directed self-learning (including digital learning) and making the most of informal, opportunistic reflective learning moments. Chapter 10 takes an educator's perspective in exploring how a reflective approach and reflective practice might be assessed. The chapter discusses a range of assessment modalities and feedback (including written, oral and practical), their strengths and limitations, how critical reflection might be built into these and how best the assessments and feedback might be used to encourage reflection. We also examine how having reflections assessed might change the way in which learners approach reflective learning and may even undermine the intended learning outcomes.

Part 4 is focussed on broader, lifelong aspects of reflection and developing as a reflective practitioner. Chapter 11 builds on earlier chapters and considers the key role of reflection in establishing, developing and re-examining professional identity. The chapter discusses how professionals develop and re-evaluate their identities. It also considers how life events, personal circumstances and personality traits might influence identity development and how guided or more purposeful reflection might help alleviate or prevent stress or burnout. We also consider how reflection can be challenging to professional identity formation. In Chapter 12 we bring the book to a close and consider the role of reflection in training, lifelong learning and continuing professional development, with a particular focus on appraisal and revalidation processes. The chapter considers how best to compile a body of satisfactory evidence for revalidation and how to structure the appraisal to incorporate reflection. It also looks more deeply into the underpinning learning processes involved and how these can aid or inhibit reflection.

What is Reflection and Why Do We Do It?

In this chapter we look at the reasons why learners are asked to reflect and what they might expect to gain from reflective learning. We will also explore the difference between the kind of reflection that forms part of everyday life, such as thinking over the day's work while driving home, and the more structured reflective learning activities that are often asked for as part of a required syllabus or training programme. We will also describe in some detail what can be achieved by reflection and look at some techniques that will help you find ways of learning reflectively that are beneficial in helping you improve your practice.

Why are Learners Required to Reflect?

Many learners, when they are first faced with having to incorporate reflective activities in their learning, are very uncertain what they have to do. Where they actually have to submit reflective learning work they are unclear what it should look like and, if it is to be assessed, what would gain them good marks. So what is it that causes teachers and educators to decide whether or not to include reflection among learning activities?

There are a number of reasons for encouraging (even requiring) doctors and other health professionals to reflect on their practice throughout their lives. Reflection, if well structured and supported, helps to put more responsibility for learning onto the learner. More than anything else, reflective learning activities should encourage learners to be constructively critical of their learning and their developing practice as professionals. In this context, 'critical' is not about being a theatre critic or finding fault, but it is about an unwillingness to accept, unquestioningly, what one is told as right or correct, a readiness to ask 'why' questions and an approach to developing practice that embeds learning from experience. Reflective learners should be willing to question the assumptions underlying their existing understanding and be prepared to probe their knowledge for inconsistencies and lack of congruity. The learner in a classroom

Developing Reflective Practice: A guide for medical students, doctors and teachers, First Edition.
Andrew Grant, Judy McKimm and Fiona Murphy.
© 2017 John Wiley & Sons Ltd. Published 2017 by John Wiley & Sons Ltd.

can easily be seen as a recipient of information and the teacher as the deliverer of it. However, we know that knowledge is constructed by the learner through social interaction with teachers and peers; therefore, to merely deliver information to a learner does not guarantee construction of any knowledge at all. Reflective learners on the other hand are being challenged to examine their current level of understanding and knowledge, and to see whether their current experience is compatible with this and, if not, what further activity is needed to bring them to the required level of understanding.

When someone is learning reflectively he or she is using a completely different sort of mental activity from that of sitting in a classroom listening to a teacher and (in theory anyway) absorbing factual information. Reflective learners, as well as exploring their own understanding and questioning things they are being told, are more likely to bring together current understanding with new information, and the active constructing of new or deeper knowledge is more likely to be the outcome from this kind of learning process (Ausubel, 2000). For example, if using a written journal as a method of reflecting, by writing down events and thoughts, learners are engaging in a different mental activity from just thinking them over or describing them to someone in conversation (Moon, 1999) (see Chapter 6).

Reflective learners need to think about *how* they learn as well as *what* they know. This kind of activity is often referred to as metacognition (see Box 2.1): in other words, thinking about, or managing, thinking.

Through metacognitive activity, reflective learners become aware of what they know, what they don't know and the importance of things that they need to know. They should also have a sense of how they best go about learning in a particular situation. This is likely to make their learning more purposeful and intrinsically motivated, for reasons from within themselves. Intrinsically motivated learning is more likely to be carried out with a deep approach, is more likely to be retained and is associated with a better affective quality for the

---

Box 2.1 Metacognition

What might sound like yet another piece of jargon, *metacognition* describes the activities that take place when a learner goes beyond trying to assimilate information and takes a more active role in his or her learning. Literally 'thinking about thinking', metacognitive activity may include

- recognizing how you learn,
- identifying for yourself what it is that you need to learn,
- recognizing gaps in your knowledge and skills,
- identifying why you need to know or to learn something for yourself and
- being aware of the reasons for learning something and its importance to you.

Box 2.2 Motivation and self-efficacy

The reasons *why* we are learning something might affect how well we learn it and how useful the learning is to us subsequently (Bruning, Schraw and Norby, 2011)

Extrinsically motivated learning takes place because the learner has been told he or she needs to learn something or is geared towards achieving something that will be seen by others as important. This might be on the instruction of a teacher or in preparation for an examination. Extrinsically motivated learning typically involves a surface approach and poorly integrated learning.

Intrinsically motivated learning is carried out because the learner realizes for themselves that the subject matter is necessary or important or that the subject stimulates interest or curiosity in them. Intrinsically motivated learning is more likely to involve a deep approach to learning and integration of the subject matter.

Self-efficacy is the sense each person has of his or her own ability to function in the world (Bandura, 1997). According to Dewey (1910), when learners realize that their understanding is flawed or incomplete it is their sense of self-efficacy that motivates them to put right the knowledge or understanding gap that they, themselves, have identified.

---

learner. This refers to the learner feeling more positive about the learning that has taken place. He or she may feel that the learning was more enjoyable or feel a sense of personal achievement. An increased management of learning, with the associated intrinsic motivation, results in a learner with a greater sense of self-efficacy. In other words the learner knows what he or she has learned and why he or she has learned it and has a good judgement of the level of his or her understanding and competence (see Box 2.2).

The Place of Reflection in Professional Development

As a medical student or qualified doctor you might find yourself asking the question 'Why am I being asked to provide evidence of reflective learning?'. When doctors were first required to participate in continuing professional development they were mainly required to attend a fixed number of hours of didactic teaching each year. However, research failed to demonstrate that this approach results in much change, less still improvement, in patient care (Mathers, Mitchell and Hunn, 2012). Over recent years, there has been a shift in the requirements for qualified, practising doctors and subsequently for medical students. For example, in the United Kingdom, as part of the annual appraisal cycle and the five-yearly revalidation programme required by the General Medical Council, every registered doctor is required to provide evidence of reflective learning activity in relation to all aspects of their work (see Chapters 11 and 12). By participating in reflective learning, practitioners are encouraged to think about incidents relating to their practice that have, in some way, been out of the ordinary and stimulated them to revisit their knowledge, skills or professional behaviours in this area. By replacing the 'hours of lectures' or conference attendance (which can easily become a tick box activity) approach with a reflective one, doctors are being asked to take a far bigger part in the ongoing management of the knowledge and skills they need to continue to practise competently and safely. Each individual practitioner will have a unique collection of knowledge and skills in relation to his or her clinical practice. Therefore, by encouraging practitioners to identify the strengths and weaknesses of their knowledge and skills base, they are more likely to undertake specific, intrinsically motivated learning activities chosen to meet their individual learning needs. When doctors attend didactic sessions or conferences, they should reflect on how they have applied what they learned in their practice.

Everything said so far applies to medical students' and doctors in training's learning as much as it does to the continuing professional development of qualified doctors. Additionally, by making reflection a part of everyday practice early in their education and training, a skill is being acquired that will help them continue to learn, grow and monitor their readiness for practice throughout their careers. However, the spirit in which doctors and medical students undertake reflection makes a massive difference to how much they benefit from it. A doctor who reluctantly completes the required elements of their portfolio for appraisal the night before the closing date for submission thinking that this is just a 'tick-box exercise' is unlikely to gain a great deal from the process. Such doctors are also likely to reinforce their view of reflective learning as not beneficial or relevant to them.

FAQ 2.1 *Is reflective learning different from what I do every day in idle moments?*

The answer to this is 'yes'.
Although reflective tasks that learners are required to do vary a great deal, here are a few ways in which they differ from the kind of reflection that everyone does, often thinking to themselves, about occurrences in their lives.

1) Most reflective learning tasks will require you to produce some form of evidence that reflective learning has taken place. This may be in the form of an e-portfolio or a reflective journal (see Chapter 9).
2) Reflective learning tasks often start by asking you to write down your experiences and actions, because this will encourage you to process (think about more deeply and in different ways about) the learning material.

3) While 'idle' reflection alone might be unfocused, reflective learning tasks will encourage you to identify outcomes such as
   a) gaps in your learning
   b) areas where you need to study
   c) changes in your understanding
   d) different ways in which you will approach things in future.

John Dewey's Contribution

Dewey's work provides the theoretical underpinning for a lot of reflective learning work that is carried out to this day. In his book entitled *How We Think* (1910) Dewey noted that reflection (as in reflective learning) is a conscious and deliberate act that begins when learners recognize that something within their understanding is incorrect or incomplete and ends when they have addressed this shortcoming.

More generally, when someone is formally reflecting on their learning, they will use some structure to write an account or to describe something that has occurred during the learning and will then address it using a set of questions or tools, for example e-portfolios with or without specific templates (see Chapters 4, 5 and 6). Although this type of reflection is similar to whenever we reflect on a particular event, what is different is that this reflection is structured around an event for a particular purpose, such as the submission of a reflective learning episode for an e-portfolio, written assignment or critical-incident or significant-event analysis. Many but not all reflective learning tasks follow this formula. We will come back to Dewey and what followed on from his work in Chapter 3, but a key point is that reflection as seen as a *deliberate* act, and therefore, to encourage such deliberation, reflective learning tasks often involve a written account of an event and a reflection on it.

FAQ 2.2 *Do I have to write this down? Is it important?*

Without writing down, or taking the time to process, the event that is being reflected upon, it is much less easy for the learner to tease out what the learning points are and what has been revealed. Jenny Moon describes the task of writing about an episode for reflection as 'explaining it to the page' (Moon, 1999).

What can be Achieved by Reflection?

As discussed earlier, reflection can help learners to increase their awareness of prior and current understanding and competence and how they can integrate this with new knowledge, skills and experiences. Through increasing awareness of their learning needs, learners can make sure that their learning is intrinsically motivated. For example, when medical students are required to reflect, as well as changing the way that they learn and the way that they process information, they might also consider some of the challenges of being a medical student, of becoming a doctor and issues about their emerging professional identity. Medical students spend a lot of time in an environment where they are, initially at least, peripheral participants in the clinical community of practice (Lave and Wenger, 1991). As students develop more competence they become more centrally involved in the practice of the community. During this time, one way in which medical students learn is by observation of qualified doctors at various levels of experience and seniority. Reflecting on learning within this medical community of practice can help students to identify the medical knowledge and clinical skills they need and, by observing the clinical practice of other members of the community, appropriate professional behaviours and approaches. For example, after observing a senior doctor dealing particularly sensitively with giving bad news to a patient, or seeing two practitioners work collectively to provide better care to a patient than either could do on their own, reflection might help students to identify what it is about the behaviour of those people that they might like to emulate in their own practice.

Part of life for every medical student and doctor is to have to deal with situations that are pressurized, stressful and emotionally difficult. Reflection, particularly if it is supported by membership of a reflective learning group with suitable ground rules (see Chapter 7), helps practitioners to deal with these situations as they occur and to identify their coping strategies and personal reserves that will help them to deal with similar situations in the future. Such reflection has been incorporated in broader health service initiatives such as Schwartz Centre Rounds®. Schwartz Rounds are regular forums for all healthcare staff to discuss difficult social and emotional issues arising from patient care (Reed *et al.*, 2015). They are facilitated and open to all health or other workers involved in patient care. A guided reflective process is used during the meeting (which typically lasts about an hour) and a growing body of evidence suggests that the Rounds provide a useful place for people to reflect on the emotional impact of engaging in 'people work' (Reed *et al.*, 2015).

Getting the Most Out of Reflection

Many learners, when they are first faced with reflective learning, feel resistant towards it (Krause, 1996; Grant, 2013). Bear this in mind when first undertaking reflective learning or if asking learners to engage in it. Try to remain open minded and curious as to what you can gain from reflection until you have had an opportunity to experience it for yourself. Although the reflective learning task you will be asked to do may come in a particular format, it is worth experimenting with ways in which carrying this out are most helpful to you and your learning. If you are reflecting on a specific event it is well worth at least making a brief record of the event quickly while it is still fresh in your memory. Although the reflective learning task you are being given to do may well involve keeping a journal or a diary, it is also worth keeping a very brief record of your journey as a new reflector. This need not take very long and need not be cumbersome, but if you are learning and gradually getting the feel for reflection in learning then it will be helpful to you to look back over a period to see how you have, over time, experienced reflective learning and its benefits for yourself.

When you are using reflection in learning, and particularly when you are beginning to use reflection, it is extremely helpful both to share experiences of reflective learning with your peers and to share the experiences you have chosen to include, particularly where these involve stressful or difficult events. The reflective learning in your programme may involve participation in regular reflective learning peer groups (they may not be called this), but if not it may well be useful for you and a group of your fellow learners to set some time aside regularly to talk about your reflective learning, how you are using it and whether you are benefiting from it. However, 'for the individual learner, there will be points at which the prevailing view of the world becomes dislodged, certainty may be eroded with uncertainty, chaos becomes apparent without stability' (Brockbank and McGill, 2009, p. 65). For this reason, it is important to set some firm ground rules amongst the members of the group around confidentiality and how much will be shared. Not setting such ground rules may result in some individuals being unwilling to speak about personal or sensitive matters or some becoming upset because they feel their views are being challenged (see Chapters 7 and 11).

Box 2.3 Reflection is useful

My first key message is to not underestimate the power of reflective practice. Prior to the course I used to find reflections a 'tick box exercise' and to be perfectly honest a waste of time. I naturally reflect upon events I encounter through my clinical work and failed to see the benefit of writing down my thoughts in a portfolio. However, as I have reflected on my leadership journey, I have come to re realise that a lot of my understanding of myself as a leader and comprehension of the leadership and management theories only came when I sat down and wrote written reflections on my experiences. Reflection helped me to explore and apply the leadership and management theories to my everyday practice.

(Written by doctor in training on leadership programme.)

Summary

We finish this chapter as we began by emphasizing that learners and practitioners get the most out of reflective learning when it is undertaken with a spirit of curiosity, with willingness to be critical and challenging of assumptions, and by being open to having your views, practice or ideas changed.

3

Theoretical Underpinnings of Reflection

> This chapter takes a multidisciplinary approach to exploring and explaining reflection for medical students, trainees and doctors. It builds on Chapter 2 by taking a historical perspective to consider and explain the emergence of reflective practice in the context of major educational, philosophical and psychological perspectives, including those of Dewey, Freire, Kolb, Vygotsky, Ausubel and Schön.

Experience has to be arrested, criticised, analysed, considered and negated to shift it to knowledge (Criticos, 1993).

In Chapter 2 we introduced John Dewey and his pioneering work on reflective learning (Dewey, 1910). Dewey emphasized that reflection was a deliberate act, and also said that reflection was what made it possible to identify what had been learned in one context and to apply it in another. He called this process 'making meaning'. It is difficult to overestimate the importance of this. It means gaining the freedom to be able to unlock and apply what we already know.

On some occasions we simply do not know the answer to a problem or question, but there are many others when we have the factual information necessary but are unable to access it or apply it to certain contexts. Dewey emphasized the importance of the attitudes of the learner to accessing or applying information, noting that in order for reflection to take place the learner needs to value personal and intellectual growth. We would add the importance of developing critical curiosity as part of the search for making meaning, asking *I wonder...* questions: *I wonder why? I wonder how? I wonder what?* and so on.

Developing Reflective Practice: A guide for medical students, doctors and teachers, First Edition.
Andrew Grant, Judy McKimm and Fiona Murphy.
© 2017 John Wiley & Sons Ltd. Published 2017 by John Wiley & Sons Ltd.

Kolb

David Kolb did much to make Dewey's work applicable to millions of learners (Kolb, 1984). He developed thinking on 'experiential learning': learning strategies that sought to use reflection to help students to maximize the learning and the making of meaning from experience. His 'Experiential Learning Cycle' was designed to guide learners through the stages that would support them in the assimilation and accommodation of learning from experience (Kolb, 1984). Kolb's model (along with other models to support reflective learning) is discussed further in Chapter 4.

> Reflection in the context of learning is a generic term for those intellectual and affective activities in which individuals engage to explore their experiences in order to lead to new understandings and experiences (Boud, Keogh and Walker, 1985, p. 19).

Freire

Paulo Freire was a Brazilian philosopher and educationalist, whose ideas have influenced school education around the world. Freire believed that education had the power to emancipate people who were oppressed, and that it was through the same mechanisms, those of challenging assumptions and attitudes and changed perspectives, that he said that this could happen (Freire, 1996). Freire describes, in disparaging terms, the 'banking model' of education. This sees the learner as an empty bank account into which teachers and educational activities 'deposit' learning. This is similar to seeing learners as 'empty vessels'.

Similarly to Dewey, Freire considers that the development of learning requires active participation on the part of the learner rather than the passive 'banking' process. Seeing learners as active constructors and mediators of their learning is a social constructivist view of the learning process (see, e.g., Bruner, 1996). The attitudes of learners, their perception of what learning entails and their ability to deal with uncertainty also contribute to the level of at which particular learners are able to work. A number of authors have produced scales of increasing sophistication of learning on this basis. Although each has its own nomenclature and number of stages, they all use the following factors to determine the level of sophistication of learning (Biggs and Tang, 2011; King and Kitchener, 1994; Perry 1970):

- ability to tolerate uncertainty
- ability to apply learning in new contexts
- integration of learning from different sources.

Applying and Integrating Learning Through Reflection

Part of the process of reflection is connecting learning from different sources and making meaning: see Scenario 3.1.

Scenario 3.1

A medical student sees a patient with a goitre. When she is asked for a diagnosis or differential the first thing she suggests is thyroiditis. Thyroiditis should be included in the differential diagnosis, but towards the bottom of the list as it is much rarer than other possible causes. The student has not seen many goitres yet, so this is an understandable mistake. Her clinical tutor gets the student to revisit the examination of the patient in her mind by asking some questions. In particular the tutor asks the student if the goitre was tender and then helps the student to realize for herself, using existing knowledge (a goitre due to thyroiditis would be tender) and correct her own error.

A student reflecting after this event, for instance writing a reflective journal, should then be able to apply new understanding to past situations and better understand what was going on in the light of the newly acquired knowledge.

Vygotsky, a Russian educational psychologist, talked about learning that could be achieved by the input of a teacher (but which the learners could not achieve on their own) as taking place in the *zone of proximal development (ZPD)* (Vygotsky, 1978). For learners to learn effectively in the ZPD requires teachers to put in place activities such as questions, prompts and challenges to help the learners to apply what they already know to the topic being discussed. This is known as 'educational scaffolding', and without it learners do not have links or links that are sufficiently strong within their cognitive structure to be able to apply relevant knowledge (even though it exists somewhere in their memory). Chapter 7 discusses different types of educational activity centred around enabling reflection in this way.

Knowledge – a Constantly-Changing Network

Where learning is largely perceived as an act of committing facts to memory, analogies such as depositing facts in a knowledge bank as described by Freire (1996), filling an empty vessel or adding 'bricks' of fact to a wall of knowledge are appropriate. However, in a model where knowledge is only constructed by the learner, these models are no longer valid. The unique body of knowledge inside the mind of each individual learner has gradually been constructed step by step since he or she was born. The brain contains a highly interactive network of information, the 'cognitive structure' (Ausubel 2000). Learning interacts with and builds this cognitive structure as new knowledge is assimilated and accommodated. Let us return, for the moment, to the concept of learning as making meaning. When coming across a new piece of information, the learner first takes in the new information using the senses. This process is referred to as 'assimilation.' In order to make meaning that has relevance, the learner needs to determine how the new information fits with the knowledge already present in his or her cognitive structure. If the new information does not resonate at all with existing knowledge, then the learner can only take it on board as unrelated factual information. In this situation, the learner may be able to reproduce the information but is unlikely to be able to apply it, particularly in new settings. In many cases, however, learners are able to find existing knowledge that is relevant to the new learning. This may be a partial understanding of the learning material but may also be contextual knowledge. Even if the learner is simply aware of names, places or acronyms, these will provide links within the cognitive structure which will help to make links to the new material.

Part of the process of meaning making involves a marrying up of new and existing knowledge. This process is referred to as 'accommodation.' In order to take new learning into the cognitive structure, the learners may need to adapt their current understanding of the subject matter and/or they may need to modify the new learning. Each act of assimilation and accommodation involves learners modifying and adapting their cognitive structures, with knowledge being constantly updated and new links made within this complex network. Ausubel called these links 'hooks' for new learning, and noted that the absence of hooks caused difficulty for learners in absorbing and retaining knowledge if learned by rote (Ausubel, 2000).

The hooks are what the teacher uses in setting up the scaffolding we discussed earlier; this is when learning is linked back to earlier learning and thus reinforced: 'thinking about Mr Patel who was admitted overnight, do you remember when we discussed the consequences of nonadherence to anticonvulsants last week? What do you think you are seeing in Mr Patel's condition that could be associated with this?'. In accommodating new learning, learners may revisit prior knowledge, but during the process they may find that with their newly acquired learning they can now explain or understand a previous episode where, until now, their understanding was incomplete (an 'Aha!' 'or 'light-bulb' moment). 'Aha! Of course that explains his signs and symptoms...'.

Deep and Surface Approaches to Learning

What the previous sections of this chapter have asked you to do is to think about how you conceptualize learning and how you learn. Exploring your beliefs and your experiences will help you to identify ways of learning that will be effective and rewarding. A group of authors, often referred to as the 'Gothenburg School', carried out a number of research studies where they explored learners' approach to their learning (Marton, Hounsell and Entwistle, 1997). Clearly, the way you perceive the task of learning is highly likely to influence the way you approach it and what you are likely to achieve. Initially, they identified two approaches: surface and deep learning. Learners adopting a surface approach are more likely to try to memorize what they learn in unrelated chunks. A learner who is given a piece of text to study and who adopts a surface approach will read the text serially; that is to say, they will try to memorize the content by breaking it up into a series of sections. The learner who adopts the deep approach, by comparison, will attempt to read the text as a whole (holist approach) and try to understand the meaning that the author is conveying. Similarly to most human behaviour, approaches to learning do not occur in a binary (entirely deep or entirely surface) fashion (Marton and Säljö, 1997), and so a third category of 'strategic learner' was added. Most learners are, however, strategic. They are able to adapt their approach to their learning according to the demands of the programme or the particular task. If an assessment rewards rote learning then the strategic learner will adopt the surface approach; if it demands deeper understanding they will adopt a deep approach.

Reflection In Action, Reflection On Action – Donald Schön

Schön gave a new perspective on reflection through his research observing trainee architects as they worked and learned. He identified two quite different ways in which reflection was used in learning and in refining professional practice, which he called *reflection-in-action* and *reflection-on-action* (Schön, 1983, 1987): see Scenario 3.2.

Scenario 3.2

If a medical student examines a patient's abdomen and realizes as he does this that when he uses the edge of his index finger to palpate the liver edge as opposed to the tips of all four fingers it is much better, this is reflection-in-action. He has recognized that his technique is flawed, corrected it and recognized that the corrected method is better, all within the one task of examining an individual patient.

If, by comparison, a student taking a history from a patient thinks that she may have caused discomfort or embarrassment to the patient in some way, she may go away after the encounter, write it up in her reflective journal and possibly discuss it with her teachers or peers. She may also look at books or e-learning packages on consultation skills. Here, the reflection is after the event, when she is no longer in the clinical environment with the patient's needs to be considered. She may, of course, try out new techniques in subsequent consultations (*reflection-for-action*), but the reflection on an event is reflection-on-action. We discuss this further in Chapter 4.

The Uncertain World of Practice

We have all, at some time, experienced a situation that was very different in reality from how we had imagined it or how it had seemed from descriptions. Many students experience a surprise at how different things are when they enter the clinical environment from the way they had imagined them before or just after starting their undergraduate programme. The patients often have complex, numerous conditions; wards, emergency departments and admissions units are often extremely busy and qualified staff may have little time to guide or teach. Writing a reflective journal can help students navigate this difficult environment and a supportive dialogue or professional conversation can help this process a great deal. Such conversations may take the form of discussing experiences and expectations through a reflective group with other students with or without the presence of a facilitator. In some medical schools, students submit their written reflections and receive feedback from a teacher in the form of a 'Socratic dialogue'. This is a conversation in which the teacher (in this case) promotes active, critical and reflective thinking through prompt questions, which require the learner to think more deeply about different aspects of a situation or dilemma.

Emotional Content of Learning

Much of the content in Chapters 2, 3 and 4 is based primarily on reflection being centred around learning as a cognitive activity that involves the acquisition, integration and application of knowledge. Reflection can go much further than this. Medical students and other health professionals have to deal with stressful and emotionally demanding situations. Sometimes the clinical environment is very busy and they may find themselves being involved in life and death situations. Most students have, at some time in their training, to accept that medical practice and healthcare are, in reality, very different from how they had imagined them before coming to university. Reflection can help learners examine their developing identities as a future members of a profession and enable them to identify the characteristics that they observe in their clinical teachers that they may wish to demonstrate in their own behaviour in the future. Chapter 11 discusses the role of reflection in developing professional identity in more depth.

Summary

This chapter has taken forward some of the discussions from Chapter 2 and related these back to some learning theories relevant to the reflective process. In particular, you have seen that reflection is a complex process closely linked to how we think learning actually happens. Reflection is about making connections with previous knowledge, experiences and feelings through a structured process. We go on to look at some of the ways in which reflection can be structured and 'framed' in Chapter 4.

Frameworks for Reflection

This chapter considers a range of influential frameworks that have been, or are currently, used to structure, explain and develop reflection. The chapter describes these in terms of the contexts in which they may be helpful and considers their strengths and limitations, including the evidence base for each.

Introduction

Reflection has been defined as a 'process of thinking, feeling, imagining, and learning by considering what has happened in the past, what might have happened if things had been done differently, what is currently happening, and what could possibly happen in the future' (Rolfe, Jasper and Freshwater, 2011, p. 12). Reflection is part of reflective practice: reflecting on experience and learning that leads to a change in actions or behaviour (Jasper, 2006). Reflective practice is primarily envisaged as being at an individual level, considering the knowledge that individuals need to attain and demonstrate and how they make changes to their individual practice. However, Rolfe, Jasper and Freshwater (2011), drawing on the work of Donald Schön, point to the more political aspects of what knowledge is, what constitutes appropriate professional knowledge and who generates, defines and holds that knowledge. Schön draws a distinction between what he calls the 'hard high ground' and the 'swampy lowlands' of professional practice (Schön, 1992). 'On the hard high ground, manageable problems lend themselves to solution through the use of research-based theory and technique. In the swampy lowlands, problems are messy and confusing and incapable of technical solutions' (Schön, 1992, p. 54). Thus a reliance solely on technical rational knowledge, which includes 'the describable, testable, replicable techniques derived from research' (Schön, 1992, p. 52), has limitations in professional practice. This reflects the limitations of applying evidence-based practice in complex, paradoxical, uncertain or rapidly changing conditions. What Schön proposed was an 'alternative epistemology of

Developing Reflective Practice: A guide for medical students, doctors and teachers, First Edition. Andrew Grant, Judy McKimm and Fiona Murphy.
© 2017 John Wiley & Sons Ltd. Published 2017 by John Wiley & Sons Ltd.

practice grounded in observation and analysis of the artistry competent practitioners sometimes bring to the indeterminate zones of their practice' (Schön, 1992, p. 51). This reflects what has been discussed in Chapters 2 and 3 about the social construction, reconstruction and mediation of knowledge that happens through reflection, conversation and experience.

A key component of reflection in action is that the practitioner actively (although it may not appear to be overt) theorizes as to what may be the best course of action in solving the unique problem or reframes it as a 'problematic situation'. The practitioner *in* the situation reflects on what has been done, achieved and presented at that moment with the knowledge used at that point of action. Schön further distinguishes between reflection *in* action and reflection *on* action (1992, p. 60). Reflection on action is looking back at what happened. In doing this, the practitioner becomes more aware of the 'tacit understandings' or cultural norms and values that are associated with the repetition of the actions taken in the practice.

Schön argues that the technical–rational knowledge dominant in the 1980s continues to be dominant in contemporary healthcare. In the hierarchy of evidence (Sackett *et al.*, 1996), what might be considered appropriate knowledge for healthcare practice is that generated through research (such as randomized controlled trials and meta-analyses) and through systematic reviews of these types of evidence. In such a hierarchy, practitioner knowledge, wisdom and expert practice might be considered less important. Schön's work and Rolfe's argument is that practitioner knowledge (knowledge gained through practice) offers an alternative epistemology of and for practice. If this is accepted, then this kind of knowledge is as valuable as and complementary to technical–rational knowledge (Rolfe, Jasper and Freshwater, 2011). The key to unlock and discover this knowledge is through reflective practice, and Rolfe argues that this process is (and should be) as rigorous as research. Just like the research process, frameworks equivalent to methods in research exist that are employed to guide the reflective process. Rolfe defines these frameworks as 'specific methods or approaches that provide help and guidance' (Rolfe, Jasper and Freshwater, 2011, p. 33), which is different from the models or theories such as those of Dewey (1910) and Kolb (1984), which underpin these frameworks. In this chapter therefore we will explore some of the most influential frameworks for reflective practice. These will include those of Borton (1970), Rolfe, Jasper and Freshwater (2011) and Gibbs (1988).

Frameworks for Reflection

Kolb: Learning from Experience

The frameworks described in this chapter draw heavily on the notion of learning from experience (Kolb, 1984), which has been described in Chapter 3. To recap, Kolb developed thinking on experiential learning, that is to say learning strategies that use reflection to help learners maximize the learning and the making of true meaning from experience. His 'experiential learning cycle' (Kolb, 1984) was developed to guide learners through the stages that would support them in the assimilation and accommodation of learning from experience. These stages are concrete experience, reflective observation, abstract conceptualization and active experimentation. This cycle of experiential learning influenced the reflective frameworks described below.

Borton's Framework

In 1970, Terry Borton described what he called a 'model for process education' (Borton, 1970, p. 93) in teaching school-age children. He draws on the idea that, although we can learn from experience, a process is required to facilitate this learning. Borton's process model has three stages: 'what?' (increasing awareness), 'so what?' (evaluating intention) and 'now what?' (experimenting with new behaviour) (Borton, 1970, p. 93) (Figure 4.1).

Borton's focus was on students knowing themselves and their own concerns and processes, and his model for process education was designed to enable this. In the first stage, 'what?', the learners draw on an experience close to them and explore their responses to the experience. They describe what happened, how they felt and what actions they took or should have taken. The process begins with and is grounded in a specific experience and involves thinking about that experience actively and purposefully. The next stage is 'so what?': this is 'rational, intellectual, cognitive – a delving into the meaning of what has just happened' (Borton, 1970, p. 96). This stage involves an analysis of the event and there needs to be some critical thinking and intellectual work to make sense of the situation. Borton recommends approaching this in two ways: both analytically and contemplatively. Rational analysis can be useful, Borton argues, but some important components of an experience such as values and feelings might be crushed by such techniques and hence Borton also recommends a more relaxed contemplative approach. In the 'now what?' stage, learners are helped by their teacher to identify processes that can help them work through their concerns, such as actions, knowledge, resources, tips, techniques and understandings.

Figure 4.1 Borton's framework (Borton, 1970).

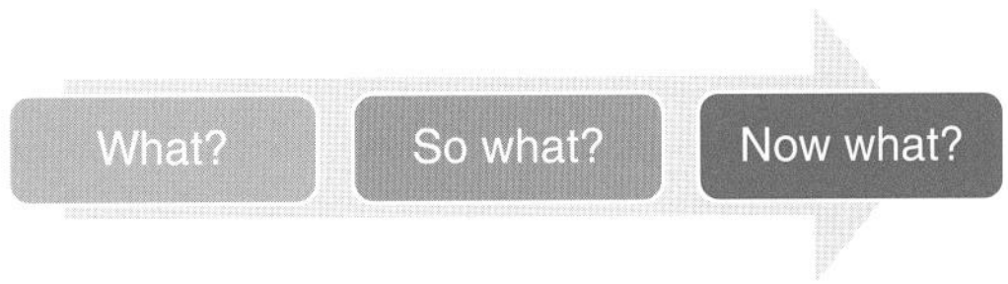

This framework is learner focused: the teacher facilitates rather than instructs. Borton writes from the perspective of an educator and so the framework is designed to help teachers facilitate learning. The three stages appear deceptively simple, but each stage contains a complexity of processes, which both the teacher and the learner have to master. This framework was very influential on subsequent frameworks for reflective practice.

Rolfe's Framework for Reflexive Practice

Gary Rolfe is a healthcare practitioner and educationalist and, in building on Borton's work, extends and develops it further into a framework that is both sequential and cyclical. Rolfe notes that the apparent simplicity of Borton's three stages might fail to provide sufficient direction for practitioners and so includes cue questions to make the process easier. In addition he expands the understanding of the 'what?', 'now what?' and 'so what?' headings. 'What?' is the descriptive level, 'so what?' is about theory and knowledge building and 'now what?' is the action-oriented reflexive level of reflection (Rolfe in Rolfe, Jasper and Freshwater, 2011, p. 45). 'Now what?' might also be referred to as 'reflection *for* action'.

Underpinning this framework is the idea of a sequence and a cycle. Practitioners at the descriptive level of reflection can benefit from describing what happened in a structured way. In this framework though, there is the opportunity to move to Level 2, which is the theory and knowledge-building aspect of reflection. Earlier, we talked of Schön's critique of technical–rational knowledge and Rolfe's assertion of the importance of practitioner knowledge gained through experience of practice. This second stage in Rolfe's framework is to identify what knowledge was actually used and what knowledge could be used in all its different forms. The analysis moves beyond considering just technical–rational knowledge to all the different kinds of knowledge that did or might inform the understanding of the situation. For example, there might be an ethical dimension to a situation, so exploring beliefs and values might also be informative.

The third level is reflexive and action orientated and forms part of the cyclical aspects of the framework. It aligns with Kolb's 'active experimentation' phase of the experiential learning cycle. The practitioner, having learned from the situation, hypothesizes what might work next time if a similar situation arose, and then tries out these actions. This active process of learning from, trying out and reflecting again on these new actions leads to theory building and knowledge generation. These theories and knowledge are grounded in practice rather than being formally 'learned'. This stage also reflects Giddens' work on social theory, where he suggests that in the late modern world individuals continually develop their self-identity through reflexivity and a reflexive understanding of their own biography (Giddens, 1991). Giddens suggests that we treat our identities as a project which, whilst having continuity, is continually reshaped and constructed in the light of experiences. In Chapter 11, we explore further how reflection and reflexivity contribute to an individual's personal and professional identity.

Borton's (1970) three key questions of 'what?', 'so what?' and 'now what?' were further developed by Driscoll (2007) in developing processes for clinical supervision in healthcare. As in the work of Borton, the process begins with a concrete experience, and as this model was designed to facilitate clinical supervision the concrete experience is usually a clinical encounter with a patient, client or peer. Similarly to Rolfe, Jasper and Freshwater, to further facilitate the use of this framework, Driscoll identified some 'trigger' questions to stimulate ideas to complete the cycle. Through the facilitative process of clinical supervision, the focus here is to learn from clinical experiences and to take actions to change practice should a similar situation arise.

Gibbs: Learning by Doing

An influential framework used extensively in education and healthcare education is that developed by Graham Gibbs (Gibbs, 1988). Gibbs is an educationalist and thus the framework is firmly grounded in learning from experience. It draws on the ideas of Dewey (1933) and Kolb (1984) in emphasizing the need to reflect and think about an experience to learn from it. Gibbs' framework (Figure 4.2) is cyclical and has six stages: description, feelings, evaluation, analysis, conclusion and action plan.

1) *Description – what happened*. This cycle begins with a concrete experience, as Gibbs believes that learning must come from some kind of experience. As it might not be enough simply to experience something to learn from it, a more active process needs to be set in place. The framework is designed to facilitate this process.

   In common with Borton's 'what?' stage, Gibbs advises us to simply describe what happened, not to make any judgements or come to any conclusions (Gibbs, 1988). In this descriptive stage, it can be useful to try to identify a single event that has boundaries around it, for example just one encounter with a patient or colleague, rather than trying to describe a whole day. Even with this approach, descriptions can be very complex, so it can be helpful to identify one significant issue in what happened to focus on (see Scenario 4.1).

Scenario 4.1

I had to go tell a patient that her test results had come back showing her cancer had spread. We need to do further tests, but the prognosis isn't too good. When I got to the bedside, her husband had just left and I was going to wait to tell her when he came back but she insisted on me telling her there and then. The patient got very angry and upset and I had to go get a nurse to sit with her and calm her down.

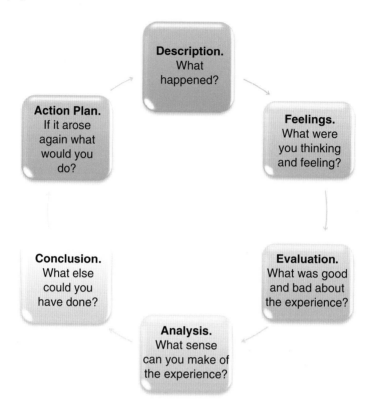

Figure 4.2 Gibbs' framework (Gibbs, 1988).

2) *Feelings.* The second stage is identifying what were the individuals' thoughts and feelings. Gibbs' work is useful in that it acknowledges the importance very early on of feelings and emotions. Significant events will generate both negative and positive feelings and Gibbs as an educator recognized the need to acknowledge these feelings in order to move on to the next stage of the cycle. If this is not done then the feelings will dominate and might be suggested to impede further learning. Gibbs advises just to list the feelings and not think about analysing them just yet (Gibbs, 1988).

Scenario 4.1 contd

I felt I'd done the best I could in giving accurate information in an empathic way
   But I was upset at the patient's reaction and angry with myself for not checking there was someone with her or getting a nurse to come with me while I told her.
   I also felt wrong-footed in not being able to take a moment to sort things out in a better way. I feel as if I've made something much worse than it was already for her.

---

3) *Evaluation.* The third stage is an evaluation, as Gibbs advises, looking for what was good or bad about the experience. It is possible to make value judgements about what happened at this stage. There might be a tendency to focus on the bad things, so it can be useful to think of what might be considered good about the experience before focusing on the bad, as not everything within an event might be bad.

Scenario 4.1 contd

I carefully prepared myself to break the news, got all the correct information and organized the next steps in the treatment plan. I could answer all the technical questions she asked. These were good aspects of the situation.

The bad aspects were really about the patient's reactions and the difficulties in managing that, compounded by the way I hadn't checked there was someone else with me or waited till her husband was back.

---

4) *Analysis.* This is a key stage and here Gibbs advises to ask what was really going on in the situation (Gibbs, 1988). In common with Borton's 'so what?' stage, Gibbs is looking for some critical thinking here in trying to make the individual stop and pause and consider the experience if possible from different perspectives. Gibbs also advises bringing in ideas and perspectives from outside the experience to aid the analysis. The benefits of reflecting in a group is that it allows these outside perspectives to be shared. Different

---

Scenario 4.1 contd

If I was the patient, I probably wouldn't have wanted to be given this uncertain (but bad) news when I was on my own, well at least, I'd have liked to have had the choice. Thinking from the patient's perspective might give me all kinds of different interpretations and explanations of what happened. The news is shattering, but they may not have understood the medical terminology, they may have felt I wasn't fully concerned, they may have had relatives who had died recently from the same condition and all these factors may have impacted on their reaction.

From my own perspective, I wonder if I was not paying sufficient attention to the needs of this patient, I think I maybe just wanted to get the jobs done and didn't think about it from the patient's viewpoint.

My action learning set was useful as they asked me whether I felt I had enough time with this patient and what training I'd had in breaking bad news. They also reminded me about some videos and training courses which offer some guidance on what I could (and should) have done in the situation.

individuals might see the situation in different ways, and this can be helpful. A bit like Borton's role of the teacher, a skilled facilitator of the group can also help the concerns to be raised and analysed and contemplated. Ideas, theories, models and knowledge from the literature can also be used to make sense of the situation.

One of the possible critiques of this framework is a lack of guidance as to what this stage of the framework entails. Alternatively, as it can be interpreted very broadly, this is a strength, in that it does not constrain the individuals to analyse in a particular way and they have the freedom to do as they wish. Regardless of how it may be interpreted, this framework is pushing the individual towards a thorough analysis of what may or may not have been happening in the experience.

5) *Conclusions.* Having analysed the situation, this fifth stage of Gibbs' framework is what can be concluded, which also links with Borton's 'so what?' stage. Gibbs suggests thinking of the conclusions at two levels: first in a general sense and second at an individual level.

Any conclusions reached will, it is hoped, be more informed, as the framework deliberately slows the reflective thinking down so that the conclusions reached are more considered.

Scenario 4.1 contd

There might be some general implications as to how the ward is organized in terms of providing time and resources to support patients receiving bad news. Also when we do this is important and this can be discussed with the nurses and ward manager.

For myself, I need to update my training on breaking bad news and work with other senior doctors to learn from them and get feedback on my own rapport and empathy.

---

6) *Action plan.* The sixth and final stage, having (hopefully) learnt from the experience, is considering what would be done next time a similar situation arose. Would things be done differently or the same? Gibbs' framework is overtly about action, as the reflective process in this framework is incomplete without stating an action plan. Implicit within this is the notion of learning from that experience in order to inform actions.

Gibbs' framework has been extensively used in healthcare curricula, as it provides an accessible framework, which guides learners through the process, resulting in an action plan for their future practice as well as identifying learning needs. The analysis section can be completed quite simply or it can be a very complex analysis of the situation. Another worked example of the use of Gibbs' model is in Chapter 5.

Scenario 4.1 contd

My action plan includes

- watching the videos on breaking bad news,
- asking my registrar to come with me next time and give me feedback afterwards,
- talk to the nurses about the best times to give bad news and ask if it's OK to work with them to make sure relatives are there,
- thinking about things much more from a patient's perspective and
- asking for help if I feel out of my depth.

Summary

In this chapter, three frameworks for reflection (Borton, 1970; Rolfe, Jasper and Freshwater and, 2011; Gibbs, 1988) have been described. Each of these frameworks considers learning from experience as central, and each proposes a framework to help individuals learn from experience through reflecting on it. These frameworks are sequential or cyclical, implying some kind of forward movement in the reflective process. All have an emphasis on learning and knowledge for clinical practice, with an expectation of action to improve practice should a similar situation arise again. These frameworks, although appearing facilitative and flexible, are designed to offer some structure to enable the reflective process to be as rigorous as possible.

It has not been possible to describe all the available frameworks, as many have been developed. Many online resources on frameworks for reflective practice exist, some of which are listed at the end of the book. It is important to remember though that frameworks are just guides to the reflective process, and the choice of a framework is therefore an individual one.

Part II

Learning Reflection

5

Reflecting in Practice

The first part of the book presented some theories and models underpinning the reflective process, proposing that reflection can and should be an important part of learning. This chapter shifts the focus to considering practical things that can be done to help reflection in clinical practice. A range of activities are suggested here. Depending on the situation and your experience, different activities might be more relevant; none is considered to be 'better' than the others, they are just different ways of helping reflection in and on practice.

This chapter focuses particularly on reflection *on* action: looking back at an experience to see what may be learned and what may be changed next time. An important part of the reflective process is to capture the experience ready for analysis, and the first part of the chapter identifies some rapid techniques for capturing clinical practice experiences. The second part provides an other example of how Gibbs' (1988) model may be used to analyse an experience from practice.

As a reminder, reflecting *in* action (or practice) is when the practitioner is in the middle of a situation and needs to appraise what is going on to select the most appropriate course of action. For experienced practitioners, this process can be very rapid as they draw on all their previous experience and make a decision in that moment. Later on, they may reflect *on* the action they have taken. For less experienced practitioners, reflecting in action is often less rapid and the appropriate response and course of action might not be entirely clear in the moment: hence the importance of reflecting *on* the action at a later date to try to learn from the experience.

Capturing and Describing the Experience

The reflective process begins with an experience that needs to be captured in some way, thus the early stages of most reflective models and frameworks focus

Developing Reflective Practice: A guide for medical students, doctors and teachers, First Edition.
Andrew Grant, Judy McKimm and Fiona Murphy.
© 2017 John Wiley & Sons Ltd. Published 2017 by John Wiley & Sons Ltd.

on capturing the experience to enable it to be described and analysed. Usually the individuals are asked to identify and reflect on something that has happened to them and, although this event can be good, bad or indifferent, the key thing is that it is of some significance to them. Students or doctors in training are often asked to select, describe and analyse a 'critical incident' or 'significant event' from their practice, although note that different institutions, specialities and programmes use different terminology (Grant 2013). It is often a situation that may be perplexing, or that causes to you think hard about what happened, so it does not have to be an action-packed or dreadful situation.

Although such experiences are usually memorable to the individual, a good habit to get into is to record them. Traditionally this has been through writing them down, but it may not be possible to start writing lengthy descriptions when in practice. The flexibility of mobile or web-based technologies provides alternative ways to capture the experience quickly, from 'less than a minute' to up to five minutes.

'Less than a Minute' Techniques

Voice Recordings

You can use a mobile phone or other device to dictate and record what has happened. This can be done very soon after the experience has occurred and then can be written down later if required. Although it is a quick technique there are some drawbacks. These chiefly relate to privacy and confidentiality, in that patient and other details may be heard by someone else if they access your phone or other recording device. Care needs to be taken that confidential details (such as patients' names or identifying details) are not recorded.

The Reflective Selfie

This is a visual way to record your experience based on your facial expression. At the end of a day in practice you take a picture of yourself with the facial expression that sums up the day and make a brief note explaining your 'selfie'. A series of these can be taken over a placement or rotation to help pin down trends in what was good or bad about that day and what could be done to make it better. It can be constructive to record your placement in this way over a period of time to see how experiences flux and change. It is also helpful to record what triggered the feelings, then when there is more time to identify what has been learned and what might need to change.

Emoticons ☺

An even quicker way is to use emoticons to summarize the day or the experience. Again record them over the whole placement or rotation and try to identify why it was a good, bad or indifferent experience for you. Like the reflective selfie, this helps to record patterns of feelings over a time period as well as recording the triggers for these feelings. It can be a useful way to help sum up a whole clinical rotation.

Word Whips

Another quick technique is 'word whips' (generationOn, 2011), where you are asked to think of one word to describe your day. Like the reflective selfie and the emoticon, this technique, although useful for capturing the immediacy of your experience and feelings, might need to be expanded upon at a later stage.

These kinds of quick technique are useful for recording trends across a period of time, summarizing an experience in reflecting both in and on practice, and might help to recall a situation. Often situations in clinical practice are very complex, and these quick techniques mean that you can focus on the most immediately important aspect for you, which you can then reflect on further at a later date. The limitation of these techniques is that they may not adequately capture the complexity and detail of the experience and provide the opportunity to explore resulting issues.

One to Five Minute Techniques

These 'less than a minute' techniques can quickly capture aspects of the experience to begin the reflective process. The activities in this next set take between one and five minutes (adapted from Jasper, 2006) and help provide more detail about the event to enable recall of the experience.

The 'Three a Day' Technique

In this technique, three key things that have happened that you feel are important are written down. This could be during the day as they occur, or at the end of the day. There are no expectations of what kinds of thing should be recorded; the important thing is to get them recorded to enable a more in-depth reflection later.

The Credit Card Technique

In thinking back on the experience, enough detail is written to fill a credit card. This takes a bit more practice, as it is important to think about the important issues before starting to write. Again, this technique is intended to avoid the need to write laboriously and should provide a concise account of the experience.

Time Limited

This is much more spontaneous, in that whatever comes to mind is written down for five minutes without stopping. There is no need to worry about spelling, punctuation, grammar or whether it appears to make any sense. It can be written in any order or in any way. Again, this provides an alternative to having to write lengthy descriptions and gives a starting point to begin your reflective thinking about the experience.

In Scenario 5.1, an example of a published critical incident is provided, which describes some significant events and experiences that happened to a doctor whilst working in a clinical area (Brady, Corbie-Smith and Branch, 2002).

Using a 'less than a minute' technique, this incident might be captured and represented as an emoticon:

The 'three a day' technique would mean identifying the three key issues and very briefly summarizing them into bullet points. For this scenario this might be

- too many serious emergency admissions
- patients dying
- physically and emotionally exhausted.

Scenario 5.1 Less than a minute and one to five minute techniques

When I was in the MICU, I was called by cross-cover to evaluate a patient for transfer. She had a slightly altered mental status and was hypotensive… We were giving her fluids, blood, pressors; it was around midnight. I got another admission and went to the ER to start seeing him. The first patient coded, and I went to take care of her again. It was a terrible, endless, isolated night. I went back to the ER to see the new admission, and another code was called. I went to that. I was the only resident who responded. The patient died…

The next morning on rounds, my attending asked me how many had survived. He said we didn't need to talk about any that had died… It was a hellish night of nearly unbearable stress and in the morning it was never acknowledged, as if it had never happened, as if my patients had never existed… What bothers me most about it was that I felt completely flat. They were dead and I didn't feel anything at all (Brady, Corbie-Smith and Branch, 2002).

Finally, if the credit card technique is used, then the key points for the individual are identified and the summary (although concise) is expanded:

Terrible night on MICU and ER. Too many admissions, patients seriously ill and died. Felt really stressed. In the morning Dr (name) didn't ask me one thing about the patients who had died and all the work I had done. <u>Worried that I couldn't feel bad that patients had died.</u>

All these techniques serve to try to capture the experience in a meaningful way for the individual as the first stage of the process of reflection.

Analysing the Experience

Having captured the experience, the next step is to analyse it. Often you will analyse and reflect on the experience yourself by thinking back on what happened, identifying the key issues or areas and then trying to make sense of it yourself. However, if you are on a course or programme that is preparing you for professional practice, you may also be required to participate in the reflective process with others (see Chapter 7). For example, you may be allocated a clinical supervisor or mentor to work on a one-to-one basis with you. You may be expected to participate in group activities with fellow learners in which incidents from clinical practice are analysed. In this case, you will be asked to present a description of a critical incident or significant event from practice along with an analysis of this event. Using a reflective framework or model can be helpful to structure your description and analysis (see Chapter 4). As in Chapter 4, we will use Graham Gibbs' (1988) reflective framework (Figure 5.1) to structure your thinking about the event from practice described in Scenario 5.1.

Description: What Happened?

This is the first stage of Gibbs's model. We need something to reflect on and that comes from experience. You may have captured what happened using some of the quick techniques described above, but often it can be helpful to provide a more detailed account of the experience. To develop the description of the experience further, Jasper (2013) recommends using the 'six wise men' approach: cue questions to develop the account of the incident more fully and ensure that all key details are captured in the description. The six wise men are who, what, where, when, how and why (Jasper, 2013).

Activity 5.1 Describing

In the incident in Scenario 5.1, use the cue questions to identify the 'who, what, where, when, why and how' of the incident.

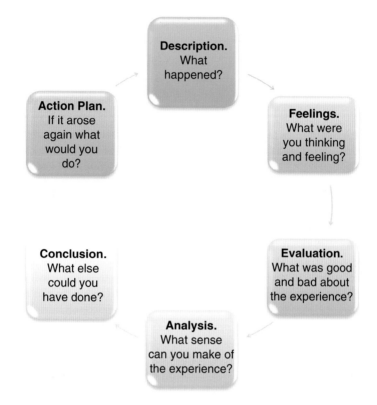

Figure 5.1 Gibbs' reflective cycle.

Feelings: What Were You Thinking and Feeling?

In Gibbs' model, this next stage is to identify the feelings that the person experienced. This offers a different dimension from experiential learning cycles such as Kolb's (Kolb, 1984). Significant events from practice are often accompanied by strong emotions, and it is important to say what these are to enable the analysis. From the example in Scenario 5.1, we can only speculate how this person might have felt, but it is useful to try to imagine how you might have felt if you were in this situation. The author uses words such as 'hellish', 'isolated', 'unbearable', 'stress', 'flat', which give strong clues as to what the predominant feelings were. When we reflect, it is important to identify (if only to ourselves) how the experience made us feel so that we can get to the root of analysing what might be going on. This is where having some distance (in terms of time) from the incident can give some perspective and help us be more objective and dispassionate, even if at the time we felt very strongly about what happened.

Activity 5.2 Feelings

What kinds of feelings might you have felt after an experience such as this?

Evaluation: What Was Good and Bad About the Experience?

The third stage in Gibbs' model is evaluation, which involves making some kind of judgement of what was good and/or bad about the experience. It can be very hard sometimes to try to identify the good things about difficult, upsetting or disturbing experiences, but there will be some and it is important to think what these might be. Surgenor (2011) suggests some key questions, which might help to evaluate the experience. These are set out in Table 5.1, along with some possible responses to them relating to this incident.

An evaluation can often be strengthened by discussing this with trusted others, who can offer different perspectives and insights on the experience than your own views.

Activity 5.3 Evaluation

From your perspective, write down what you consider from the incident might be the good and bad, positive or negative aspects of this experience. For example, it might be the readiness of this doctor to continue to respond when each emergency call was put out, a more negative aspect is possibly how burnt out and exhausted the doctor felt.

Analysis: How Can I Make Sense of This Experience?

This next stage of Gibbs' model is when even more questions start to be posed and the experience is unpicked into all its components. Experiences are usually very complex, raising many challenging issues. One technique to use is to try

---

Table 5.1 Evaluation.

What went well?	Very difficult to see any things that well. Did go down promptly to see the patients.
What did you do well?	Gave the right treatments and did the right things.
What did others do well?	Not sure
What went wrong or did not turn out how it should have done?	The patients died despite efforts. My physical and mental efforts were not recognized.
In what way did you or others contribute to this?	Senior doctor not recognizing all the effort made and the patients' deaths as not significant.

to clearly identify the one aspect about the incident that feels very important and then focus on this for the analysis. This will vary from individual to individual. For example, in the incident in Scenario 5.1, the author ends with the statement 'What bothers me most about it was that I felt completely flat. They were dead and I didn't feel anything at all'. This lack of feeling could be the significant issue for the person in this account.

Once the significant issue has been identified, the next step is to analyse it further. Breaking an issue down into all its component parts to make sense of it can be complex. 'Thought clouds' or linear thinking are useful techniques where the significant issue is posed and then the many different questions and issues allowed to emerge (see, e.g., Figure 5.2).

As you can see from the initial question, 'why did I stop feeling?', more questions and issues arise, and it is at this point that the individuals will need to seek answers to their questions. It is possible to carry out this process alone, but a group, mentor or supervisor can be very helpful in helping you to think about the issue in different (possibly unexpected) ways. Other answers might come from sources such as research, theories and online resources, and your supervisor or facilitator might steer you towards some of these.

In the incident in Scenario 5.1 many complex issues exist, but in Figure 5.2 we focussed on the identification of the significant issue 'why did I stop feeling?'. Posing this question might lead to thinking about several explanations for why the individual might stop feeling emotions in his or her practice. One possible explanation is the idea of 'burnout', so the next set of questions posed in this analytic process might be 'what is burnout?', 'what causes it?', 'how might it be recognized?' and 'what can be done about it?'. Trying to find the answers to these questions might lead to discussions with friends, peers, supervisors,

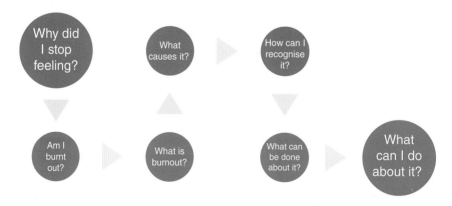

Figure 5.2 The analytical process.

mentors and lecturers and looking at the theoretical literature or websites. For example, Maslach (1982) is a key author in the description of the burnout syndrome and in developing tools to measure burnout. 'Burnout is a syndrome of emotional exhaustion, depersonalization and lack of personal accomplishment that can occur among individuals who do "people work" of some kind' (Maslach, 1982, p. 3). The first component of his burnout syndrome is emotional exhaustion, where the individual feels drained and unable to face the emotional demands of others. To cope, the individual cuts off from emotional engagement and appears detached. With increased detachment comes the appearance of indifference and coldness, which is characteristic of the second component of depersonalization. Now the worker may expect the worst of others and actively dislike them. These negative feelings towards others can then be turned into negative feelings about the self, in that the individual is now aware that he or she has turned into someone that nobody likes, and a feeling of reduced personal accomplishment results. This is the third component of burnout, and the individual begins to doubt if he or she is right for the job. Understanding burnout leads to an awareness of strategies that the person might carry out at both an individual and an organizational level to offset the effects of burnout.

Burnout is just one way of providing an explanation of the issues within this event, and other ideas or explanations may be more useful or relevant. The important thing is that the individual is not stuck at this point, the reflective process moves him or her towards learning more about what has been discovered and making changes.

Activity 5.4 Analysis

Burnout has been suggested here as one possible way to analyse this experience. What other possible explanations are there?

Conclusion

Having completed the analysis, the next stage of the model asks the following questions.

- What could have been done differently?
- What has been learned from this experience?
- What has the analysis told you?

It may be that the analysis has generated some knowledge and insights so that for example the individual recognizes burnout, what causes it and importantly what could be done to reduce the effects of burnout on him or her as an individual.

Action Plan

In the action planning stage, the individual needs to identify what he or she might do next time if a similar situation arose or what action he or she needs to take to learn more. Depending on the situation, it may be that the same course of action or a different course of action might be taken. In Figure 5.2, the issues and questions raised were around burnout and therefore the action plan would include the individual looking at ways to protect him- or herself from the effects of burnout. It would be critical here to think about and summarize what has been learnt from reflecting on the significant event and, even more importantly, what needs to be learnt for the future.

Activity 5.5 Action planning
If a similar situation arose, what different actions could be taken?

Gibbs' model was devised for use in education, and one of its limitations is that it does not fully allow an action plan for clinical practice settings (Jasper 2013). Being aware of a range of models and frameworks can be helpful to overcome such limitations. As an example, in Chapter 4 the work of Borton (1970) was described. This is a deceptively simple model incorporating three stages: *what? so what?* and *now what?*. It is the *now what?* (the plan for action) that is so important here. This is when new approaches are derived, the consequences of these are explored and awareness is raised of wider contextual issues and possible actions to deal with these. In the incident analysed in this chapter, the discussion might move to considering wider factors beyond those of the actions of the individual and what they may be able to influence, for example the following questions.

- Are there enough doctors rostered to cover night shifts?
- Who makes these decisions and on what basis?
- Can these decisions be challenged?
- What about the support and supervision of doctors in training?
- Was this a one-off incident or is it characteristic of a culture in which supervision and support may be lacking?

Part of the reflective process is to move beyond the individual experience to consider the wider context and how that impacts on the individual's experience. It begins with the individual experience but can move to considering much wider issues. In Chapter 8, we look in more depth at the process of critical thinking in which the individuals become aware of the context in which they provide care and how this impacts on their individual practice.

Summary

In this chapter we have looked at some techniques for quickly capturing practice experiences ready for describing and analysing them, and provided an example of how a practice incident might be analysed using Gibbs' model of reflection.

6

Writing Reflectively

> In this chapter, writing as part of the reflective process is explored in more depth; we will define reflective writing and look at two different types of reflective writing: personal and informal reflective writing, and more formal reflective writing, which might be part of course requirements.

What is Reflective Writing?

As we have noted previously, the reflective process begins with something that has been experienced by the person or persons. This experience needs to be captured in some way, and as discussed in Chapter 5 this can be in a variety of formats, including audio and visual as well as written. As part of being on a professional practice course which includes reflection, there is an expectation or requirement to produce some kind of written account of the experience and the subsequent analysis. This is usually to demonstrate that there has been some form of learning from the situation, some appreciation that there may be a need to change some aspect of the individual's practice and evidence of critical reflective thinking. Jasper (2013) argues that reflective writing is different from other forms of writing in that it is about learning. Through the process of reflection you might come to a deeper or different understanding of the experience on which you have been reflecting. Bassot (2012) suggests that the act of writing helps to slow thought processes down and encourages deeper critical and reflective thinking.

Different Types of Reflective Writing

Jasper identified different types of reflective writing (Figure 6.1), which she divides broadly into analytical and creative. For the purposes of this chapter, this has been modified to include reflective essays and portfolio writing.

Developing Reflective Practice: A guide for medical students, doctors and teachers, First Edition. Andrew Grant, Judy McKimm and Fiona Murphy.
© 2017 John Wiley & Sons Ltd. Published 2017 by John Wiley & Sons Ltd.

Creative Writing

This kind of writing is more informal and personal and may not necessarily be seen by others. In creative writing, it is possible to be flexible and not have to follow too many rules as to how and what is written (Jasper, 2008). It can take many forms, such as poetry and stories, but these do not have to be award-winning, 'good' poems or stories. As the poem in Box 6.1 illustrates, they can be an effective way of communicating many of the complexities within a single clinical practice encounter between a patient and a healthcare professional.

The poem is based upon an experience from practice, which has been captured and recorded in this particular way. You can see the elements of description as outlined in the first stage of Gibbs' model together with some indication of the feelings felt by the person who experienced it. The poem then captures the experience, which would then provide the platform for further analysis, discussion and interpretation.

Telling a story is another creative writing technique that Jasper identified; it usually has a beginning, middle and end and a central message. Just like a poem, a story will have at its core an experience, which is then retold as a narrative. Both poems and stories have some kind of structure. If structure is inhibiting, then Jasper suggests imagining writing a letter or an email to the

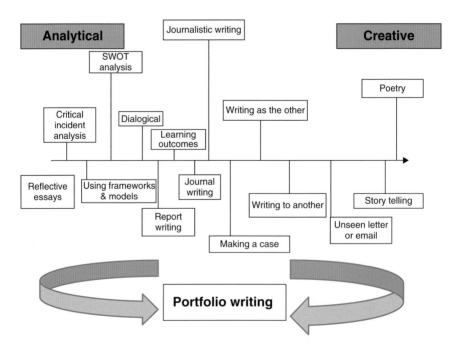

Figure 6.1 Different types of reflective writing (after Jasper, 2006, p. 89).

other person in the experience detailing the experience from your perspective, although it is never a particularly good idea to actually send it.

Another interesting technique is to try to imagine that you are the other person in the story. For example, in the poem *The Ward Round* (Box 6.1), you could imagine this experience from the perspective of the doctor or the ward sister. This provides a different angle on the experience and therefore would frame the analysis in a different way. You could (as Jasper suggests) 'make a

---

Box 6.1 Example of creative writing – poetry

The Ward Round
The doctor comes to see Nellie.
The sister stationed at her head looks on.

We need to fit a catheter, the doctor says.
What de yer want to do that for? Nellie asks.

A catheter is a device we fit…
he starts to explain

I know what one is, she interrupts
I might be 92 but I'm not stupid!

What I want to know is -
Why yer want to fit one?

Because you smell, he says.

The sister and I lock eyes across the ward
Our open mouths a mirror image of shock.

You cheeky beggar, Nellie shouts
How dare you come in here and tell me I smell!

The doctor slams Nellie's file shut
and storms out. The sister hurries after him.

I want to cheer and whistle.
Well done Nellie!

But Nellie is not rejoicing.
She looks at me with brimming eyes,

I don't smell do I?

No Nellie, I say,
You don't smell.

Sylvia Perry (2014)

case' for the different perspectives of those involved in the situation described in the poem.

Another, possibly more objective technique, would be to imagine yourself as a journalist reporting on the situation. So how might a journalist observing the encounter between Nellie and the doctor on the ward round report it? Journaling apps and online blogs, which throw open personal thoughts and experiences to the whole world, are available on the Internet. An example of an online blog describing an incident from practice is given in Box 6.2. In this example, the experience is described and the author's feelings are identified, together with some lessons for future practice as a doctor.

These types of online posting open up private thoughts and feelings to public scrutiny and so care needs to be taken when using any form of social media. In healthcare, where patients and other staff members are involved, it is extremely important that patient and staff confidentiality is maintained and people are not identified in public when they have not consented. In the United Kingdom, the General Medical Council (GMC) (2013) publishes guidelines on the use of social media. The GMC acknowledges that they can be very useful tools for sharing thoughts and experiences with others, but they can have serious implications if they are misused. In the example of the online blog in Box 6.2, the student's identity is not revealed and neither is the identity of patient or the hospital. So think carefully about the medium as well as the purpose of any reflective diary or journal.

Box 6.2 Example of an online blog

a letter to my dying patient. http://mylifeasamedstudent.tumblr.com/

Dear Ms B,
We didn't know each other well. You might recognise my face from rounds, I was the girl in the corner holding your numbers, looking at the ground or out the window. I occasionally asked you how you were, and you always told me the same thing – pain, so much pain. And I didn't know what to do. I wanted to hold your hand, but my head always made excuses. I had to continue on the round, I had to be professional, I had to maintain my distance. But I always thought about you through the day. I thought about how I wanted to sit by your bed and hear your stories, capture your last days on earth, capture the rich life I'm sure you lived.

I was there when your family was told the news. I saw how they reacted to your prognosis, and I wished you were awake to see it – not to see the pain your children were in, but so that you would realised just how loved you've been. I half-smiled at your son as I left the room, unsure of what to say, knowing that no words could take away his sadness, his grief, or his anger.

There's nothing I can do to cure you. I'm just a medical student, and even if I was a doctor, there's no medicine to make you better. We can make you comfortable, we can give you pills and injections and fluids and hope that you'll be peaceful. I hope you'll be peaceful. I hope that whatever awaits you on the other side is beautiful and that this illness that haunts you is gone. I hope that you can see your children and protect them as they go forth, and that you know that you were loved. You were cared for. You meant the world to someone.

I hope you enjoyed the journey. I hope that your life has been filled with smiles and joy. I hope you found a way to make the world a better place during your stay. I hope that, in your final moments, you remembered the good times, the days filled with happiness.

And you may never know this, but you made a difference to me. When I see another patient approaching their final moments, I will stop and talk. I'll ask them how they are, if there's anything they need, about their life, their children, their loved ones. I promise that I won't just be a doctor, I'll be someone who makes them feel valued. I'll make them feel that their last moments are being remembered.

I'm sorry that I didn't do that for you.

All the best,

My Life as a Med Student

These more informal ways of writing are very useful to enable the capturing and description of meaningful experiences. However, as part of a course, you might be asked to do more formal reflective writing. Here, although the writing might be creative it may need to be more structured, edited, presented and organized so as to meet the requirements and expectations of those who asked you to prepare your reflective writing. We move now towards the more analytical end of the different types of reflective writing (Jasper, 2006).

Analytical–Academic Reflective Writing

Journal Writing

Reflective writing can be captured in reflective journals and diaries, which provide a record of everyday events and experiences. Bassot (2012) identifies the benefits of keeping a reflective diary, arguing that it helps to clarify what you are thinking, is written in the moment and provides a record of your learning and development over the duration of the course.

Just as in any other diary or journal, the day's events are recorded, analysed and interpreted as desired. Diaries can be written in paper diaries or notebooks and can remain your private thoughts not to be seen by others. As part of course requirements, you may be asked to keep a 'reflective journal'. This is more than just a chronicling of events and is used to demonstrate that the learner has made a link between his or her experiences in practice and the teaching and learning provided on the course. Again, there are different techniques and styles for writing journals. The strategies in Box 6.3 are based on Bringle and Hatcher's "Reflection in service learning: Making meaning of experience" (1999), as drawn on by Sloan and Hartsfield (www.aacc.nche.edu/Resources/aaccprograms/horizons/Documents/reflection_3.pdf).

It can be seen from these examples of different types of journal that a key activity is to make connections between what has been experienced in practice

---

Box 6.3 Different types of journal style

- *Personal journals*. Learners write freely about their experience; usually done at least weekly. They might need to submit it to their teachers for review. This can be useful to record experiences which might be used as a basis for a reflective essay. (Julie Hatcher, Indiana University–Purdue University at Indianapolis.)
- *Highlighted journal*. Before learners submit the personal journal, they highlight sections of the journal that directly relate to learning outcomes that are to be achieved. (Gary Hesser, Augsburg College.)
- *Key phrase journal*. Teachers provide a list of key terms (for example 'confidentiality') at the beginning of the semester. The journal entries then provide examples of how this concept is experienced in a practice placement. (Julie Hatcher, Indiana University–Purdue University at Indianapolis.)
- *Dialogue journal*. Learners submit loose-leaf pages from a dialogue journal for the teachers to read and comment on. This can provide continual feedback to students and prompt new questions for them to consider throughout the course. (Goldsmith, 1995.)
- *Double-entry journal*. Students write one-page entries each week. On the left-hand page they describe personal thoughts and reactions to the placement experience, on the right key issues from class content and literature. Students then draw arrows indicating relationships between their personal experiences and course content. (Cross and Angelo, 1993.)
- *Three-part journal*. Each page of the journal is divided into thirds with weekly entries written. In the top third, they describe some aspect of the placement experience; in the middle, how the course content relates to their practice experience; in the last third, how the experience and course content can be applied to their personal or professional life. (Robert Bringle, Indiana University–Purdue University at Indianapolis.)

placements and what has been taught in the university setting. As part of formal academic writing for a course, the teachers are looking for these connections and also to identify gaps in the student's knowledge.

Learning Outcomes

Learning outcomes are action statements that communicate to both the learner and the teacher what the learner is expected to learn or achieve on aspects of the programme. All parts of a programme have identified learning outcomes: the programme itself, modules or units and clinical practice experiences. Learners also need to be able to identify their own additional learning outcomes. Part of the reflective process is making the connection between learning outcomes set by yourself or the organization and the teaching and learning experiences provided by the programme. The examples of journal styles in Box 6.3 illustrate different ways in which the learning outcomes might be connected to the reflective entries. Table 6.1 provides an example of a learning outcome and a reflective journal entry from James (a medical student) about his practice which demonstrates that the learning outcome was achieved.

Dialogical Writing

Jasper (2013, p.155) describes dialogical writing as a hypothetical conversation between the individual and another person, who may or may not have played a significant part in the event experienced. This can be useful in difficult situations, where the individuals might want to put their case across as to why they took the actions they did and then try and imagine how the other may respond to this case. This 'conversation' is written down, which allows the different

Table 6.1 Learning outcomes and reflective journal entries.·

Learning outcome	Reflective journal entry
Obtain a patient's history and perform a physical examination in a logical, organized and thorough manner. Adapt to the urgency of the medical situation and the time available.	It wasn't until I clerked my first patient, that I was better able to understand the consultant's behaviour. 'Just do a quick history and exam and present back to me in say 10 minutes?' I was asked by an F1. My patient was 'Harry', an elderly, mildly confused man. His story was jumbled and confused. I became impatient wanting to just extract the 'important' information from him. I tried to hurry him along mindful of the time, stopping him from telling me the 'softer' information. I was seeing the patient as a nuisance, someone that was disguising his own history from me – an obstacle to my efficiency. Almost immediately after the encounter, I began to feel terrible about how I had acted.

Box 6.4 Example of dialogical reflective writing

Me: 'almost immediately after the encounter, I began to feel terrible about how I had acted'

Ravi: 'why did you feel so terrible?'

Me: 'because I felt I'd been in such a rush to please the F1 that I forgot I was dealing with an older, vulnerable person'

Ravi: 'do you think pleasing the F1 is about doing things quickly or compassionately? You're only a second year student after all, they don't expect us to do things really efficiently yet'

Me: 'I hadn't thought until we had this conversation that I was trying to please someone. I thought I was a caring person, I'd feel horrible if someone did that to my grandfather'

Ravi: 'so how are you going to do things differently?'

Me: 'tomorrow, I'm going to see Harry and just sit and have a chat with him, listen to what he has to say. I think I'll talk to the F1 as well, she's really nice and can probably give me some ideas as to how to take histories from confused people'.

---

perspectives to be considered and analysed. This is a more technical style of writing than the writing to another, which Jasper describes as a type of creative writing. Taking the example in Table 6.1, dialogical writing might go as follows. James (the medical student) is 'me' and his (imaginary) peer student is 'Ravi' (Box 6.4).

Critical Incident Analysis

Towards the more analytical end of Jasper's continuum of types of reflective writing is critical incident analysis. Formal academic writing usually revolves around the analysis of a critical incident or significant event which the learner has experienced. The term 'critical incident analysis' is used differently by different disciplines. It was associated initially with Flanagan in 1954 in looking at analysing jobs to identify how and why they were successful. An example of critical incident analysis in this context was its use in the airline industry, where aviation 'near misses' were analysed to identify extremely good aspects and extremely bad aspects of the incident in order to inform on what should be done and what should be avoided.

Critical incident reporting is also seen in healthcare settings where a critical incident occurs, in which there may have been harm or a near miss incident with a patient. In order for the whole team to learn from this, the incident is formally reported, relevant data is collected and analysed and the results are formally fed back to the team in order that practice becomes safer. A critical

---

Box 6.5 Sample critical incident report suggested headings (http://www. monash.edu.au/lls/llonline/writing/medicine/reflective/5.xml)

1) Context of the incident
2) Details of the incident
3) Thoughts, feelings and concerns
4) Demands
5) Impact on studies.

---

incident report is therefore a very structured, objective and analytical process looking at an adverse clinical event (Mahajan, 2010). In an educational context, you might be asked to produce a critical incident report reflecting on your progress through the course. Box 6.5 provides some headings that may help to structure such a report.

Reflective Essay

In a reflective essay (which may vary in length between 400 words and up to 3000 words on some programmes), you will be required to write about, describe and analyse something from your own experience in practice. A number of models exist:

- you may be asked to identify and analyse one incident or significant event from your practice in depth (see above);
- another model is where you are asked to describe your 'learning journey', for example to look back at your development from when you started a programme to the end and highlight key learning points;
- some reflective essays are structured around some key questions that learners are asked to reflect on and respond to, for example 'from your experiences in working in multi-disciplinary teams, what are some of the issues you've observed and encountered?';
- others are structured around a number of key learning events, for example your first patient encounter, first death, leading a team etc.

Whatever the model, all reflective essays involve using some kind of model or framework, such as those described in Chapter 4, to give them some structure. In the reflective essay, the student draws on his or her own personal experience, seeks to explain and interpret that experience and then looks to some of the various theories in the literature or areas that have been formally taught to further explain and interpret. The 'triangulation' of observation/experience and the literature is a key element of assessed reflective practice. In this way, it is hoped that new insights and learning might occur. On your programme, guidelines might be given to you on reflective writing and you may be asked to use one of the models outlined in Chapter 4, such as Gibbs (1988) or Rolfe, Jasper and Freshwater (2011). These models usually provide a framework for how to structure your reflection, but regardless of what kind of model you might use in formal academic reflective writing there are usually the following key elements.

A Description of the Experience

This will usually be written in the past tense, as you are reflecting *on* action. It is also acceptable when recounting the experience, to use the first person, i.e. 'I felt that…'

Interpretation and Analysis

You will be offering your own (and possibly other) interpretations of the experience, as well as an acknowledgement of your own (and possibly others') feelings. You might be expected to use the literature and the theory you have been taught on your course to further aid your interpretation and analysis of the experience you have described.

An Outcome

In formal academic, reflective writing, your assessors probably want to see three key things: first, that you have learned. You have connected your own personal experience with some of the literature and theories that you have been taught or have identified yourself. Second, they want to see that having learned something this will have a positive effect on your future practice, so this is where *reflecting on (future) action* is important. Finally, they are looking for evidence that you are developing skills as a critical thinker and a reflective practitioner. They want to see that you can analyse and interpret your practice and that of others. So the example of the online blog in Box 6.2 would partially meet their expectations. The experience is well described and the feelings are well captured, but for formal academic writing further analysis, interpretation and learning from that experience would be required. Your reflective writing should demonstrate (depending on what stage of a programme you are on) that you are moving up in levels: From Level 1, being that you can describe what was going on, to Level 2, showing that you are starting to identify the knowledge you used and knowledge that you could have used or might use in future, and finally to Level 3, which is an understanding of how the wider context, for example social, cultural and political factors, might shape your practice. Learning to be a reflective practitioner is an active process with skills to be learned, and reflective writing is one of these skills. Finally, although formal reflective writing is often less formal than writing an academic essay, you still need to adhere to formal conventions such as correct referencing techniques.

Portfolio Writing

As part of your programme, you may be asked to compile a portfolio. A portfolio is literally a case containing papers, drawings or maps. You have a portfolio of investments if you are in finance or a portfolio of responsibilities if you are a minister of state. In professional practice, a portfolio usually involves a systematically assembled collection of key content that helps to demonstrate that you have the required skills, competencies, attitudes and attributes to be able to perform your job. Portfolios often have reflective elements within them, usually in the form of a critically reflective narrative or commentary that highlights the connections between these assembled objects (or evidence) to show that you have met the required learning outcomes. So, for example, if you went on several visits to different clinical placements and had a record of these visits and a report from your clinical supervisor or preceptor, then the reflective narrative would pull these together and demonstrate what you had learned from these various placements as a whole, showing your progression and further learning points.

Portfolios can be presented as written documents but increasingly are presented electronically as e-portfolios. This allows more flexibility and creativity in presenting the portfolio, which can include a range of media not just written text. Your portfolio may consist of some of the elements described in this and Chapter 5 to provide examples of the reflective process. It could include reflective selfies, emoticons, voice recordings, video diaries and other visual images. Key articles can be uploaded and included alongside elements such as a SWOT analysis and entries from reflective e-journals. If your portfolio forms part of a programme, you should be provided with guidelines as to what might be included.

Some Issues with Reflective Writing

Some evidence exists (Grant, 2013) that reflective writing is (at least initially) seen as a pointless chore, as a distraction from the 'real' work of learning that is really needed to graduate successfully. There is some evidence however that having to think and write about practice can be beneficial to learners in getting under the surface of what is happening for them in practice. Even straightforward descriptions can, after analysis, reveal sets of issues that may never have been considered before.

Learners might also feel that they are writing to a recipe that is set by their teachers and therefore censors what they are really thinking and feeling. This may happen in formal academic writing that is presented for assessment, but more informal ways of capturing and describing experiences give opportunities for less constrained reflective writing and thinking. Other learners see reflective writing as a 'tick box' exercise rather than an opportunity for some meaningful professional development. Formal academic reflective writing is often seen as very challenging, particularly when learners are trying to connect their personal experience with sets of theoretical knowledge and research (Bowman and Addyman, 2014). Teachers can help to provide structure, guidance and support for learners in writing reflectively to help address some of these issues.

Summary

In this chapter we have looked at different types of and techniques for reflective writing. Writing, reflectively or otherwise, takes practice, and using models and techniques as described can help learners to get the most out of both formal and informal reflective writing.

Reflective Activities

This chapter considers a range of face-to-face activities occurring in learning and clinical practice settings that incorporate reflection. These might involve working on a one-to-one basis with a supervisor or working in a small group of peer learners with a facilitator. Activities explored include problem- and case-based learning, supervision, appraisal, mentoring and coaching.

Types of Reflective Learning Activity

Problem-Based Learning

Problem-based learning (PBL) is a widespread learning strategy used in medical education and other disciplines. It originated in the late 1960s at McMaster University in Canada, where it was noted that the traditional instructional techniques of students attending many lectures to provide them with knowledge, in particular biomedical knowledge, was not always helpful to students solving clinical problems. PBL is underpinned by an assumption that everyday learning occurs through the solving of problems and that the problem is presented before the learning begins. Groups of students are presented with carefully constructed 'problems', with a range of resources including a tutor to help them solve the problems. There are various versions of this process, with the Maastricht seven-jump process (Gijselaers, 1995) being widely used. This was developed at Maastricht University from 1976 to provide a framework to facilitate student learning. The first step is to try to make clear unfamiliar terms and ideas. Having done this, the second and third steps are to really define what the problem is and to try to understand it through analysing it. From this analysis hopefully will come a list of possible explanations with an identification of what needs to be learnt. The sixth step is to go away and gather information to learn about these possible explanations, with the final step being to use this new knowledge to further understand and solve the presented problem.

Developing Reflective Practice: A guide for medical students, doctors and teachers, First Edition.
Andrew Grant, Judy McKimm and Fiona Murphy.
© 2017 John Wiley & Sons Ltd. Published 2017 by John Wiley & Sons Ltd.

A key characteristic of PBL is that the problem or issue is presented to the learners first before there is any other teaching. The problem is presented; the learners identify what they need to know and then actively seek out this knowledge and feed it back to their peers. PBL is not problem-solving learning, because it may not be possible to 'solve' the problem, but it is possible to learn from the problem. Nor does it require teacher-led scenarios, although scenarios are often part of the total approach.

In PBL the curricular content is organized around problem scenarios rather than subjects or disciplines. The students work in teams or groups to solve or manage these situations; they are not expected to find predetermined 'right answers'. PBL means that the curriculum needs to be based around real life, realistic issues and topics with sets of learning experiences and opportunities to help the learner make sense of the issue and learn from it.

PBL changes the role of the lecturer to a guide in the process of learning rather than a fount of all knowledge. The student becomes an active participant in his or her learning, an independent learner who is able to problem solve creatively and has learnt about him- or herself as a learner within a group. Not only do learners 'learn' material: they also develop skills to actively solve issues and the ability to retrieve appropriate information to equip them to manage the complex clinical problems they might encounter in future.

The similarities between this and the reflective processes described so far in this book are apparent. Like the reflective process, PBL begins with an issue or problem to be solved or explored with an expected outcome that some form of learning will occur. Central to this process is the need for thinking and critical thinking to frame the problem and to consider it from different perspectives to allow it to be re-framed and a solution found. Like the frameworks of reflection described in Chapter 4, analysis is needed, but, as Borton (1970) suggested, creative contemplation as well as rigorous analysis may also be required. There are also similarities in terms of approaches to knowledge types, uses and generation. Schön (1983) identified the limitations of what he called 'technical–rational' knowledge for professional practice. So in common with proponents of PBL, there was recognition that just teaching biomedical knowledge might not fully equip students to solve some of the messy problems encountered in professional practice. All kinds of knowledge, including knowledge that is gained from practice, might be drawn on to find a solution in PBL. Similarly, the reflective process, including all of the reflective frameworks described in Chapter 3, emphasizes the need to identify the knowledge that was or might have been useful in the situation.

In PBL, the focus is on learning, not necessarily teaching, in order to foster within students the capability for life-long, self-directed learning. Reflective practice also shares this as an objective in developing within individuals the capacity to reflect, think and learn independently as well as within a group.

Case-Based Learning

Another learning activity that involves the skills of reflection and critical thinking is case-based learning (CBL). This is a technique used in some medical schools in which students are presented by their teachers with a 'case' that is used as a trigger for learning. The case may be a patient scenario, a clinical case or some other trigger, such as a series of blood results for interpretation. CBL is similar to but not the same as PBL, with the main difference being that in CBL students will have some prior knowledge, which they can use to analyse the case. Thus other types of learning resource such as lectures, workshops, placement experiences and online resources will be clustered around the case to enable learning to take place. The similarities to the reflective process and learning cycles described in Chapters 2, 3 and 4 are evident here. A case is presented from clinical practice and analysed by the group. In doing this, the group identifies the gaps in their knowledge and what they need to know, with key areas of their learning identified. The group works to retrieve the knowledge needed and disseminates this back to the group as a whole, with a further identification of those areas of practice that might need improvement. In all these activities, the skills of description, knowledge connection and critical thinking, which are core to the reflective process, are also needed.

Supporting Reflective Learning

Supervision

Supervision has been defined as watching and directing what someone does and how they do it, usually with a more experienced person being the supervisor. In UK medical education, students on placement should be overseen by an 'educational supervisor' (GMC, 2009). This individual could be within the placement area or within the medical school, and should be responsible for monitoring the student's progress against relevant learning objectives. In this more formal model of supervision the purpose is to do the following.

1) Allow for discussion, dialogue and feedback around events that have happened in practice.
2) Keep reviewing the learning outcomes to ensure the student is on target to achieve these.
3) Develop and change the learning contract, with action plans to ensure the learning outcomes are achieved.
4) Explore practice issues to deepen the student's knowledge and understanding.

(Alsop and Ryan (1996) cited by McClure (2005), University of Ulster.)

The experience of supervision for the student is shaped by the supervisors themselves (Rolfe *et al.*, 2011). In one sense the supervisor's role is to 'oversee', and thus may be directive and very focused on the learning outcomes. A more reflective approach is where the supervisor and student work together to understand practice and the student's own practice. Rolfe *et al.* (2011) suggest that a combination of these two approaches helps to maximize the learning experience of students on professional healthcare courses. Both student and supervisor need to prepare for these sessions, with the student being active in identifying events from practice that are to be discussed and the areas of learning that need to be addressed and developed further. The supervisor will act as a facilitator to help the student in this process and will provide feedback on the student's performance in practice as appropriate. At the end of the supervision session, the student's progress has been reviewed, issues from practice have been discussed and an action plan for future learning and supervision sessions identified and agreed. Rolfe *et al.* (2011) also see this supervisory process and relationship as an opportunity for reflective writing together, to record the process and agree on future action plans.

To achieve this, there needs to be a good relationship between supervisor and student that is characterized by effective communication, trust and openness. This may take time to develop, and relies on both the supervisor and student being self-aware, honest and open. Both need to be able to be aware of and question their own beliefs and values and show willingness to dialogue and to be critical. For example, in Scenario 7.1 we can see how the supervisor helps James to use his reflections to develop a learning plan.

Appraisal

One element in the supervisory or line management process may be appraisal. At undergraduate or postgraduate training level, appraisal is checking performance against expected criteria such as the achievement of learning outcomes. This may be based on a self-assessment of performance by the learners in terms of how they feel they are getting on and feedback from others in the team (e.g. through multi-source feedback). In this sense, the learners may be asked to 'reflect' on their performance in practice, evaluate this performance and focus on not just perceived weaknesses but their strengths as well. Chapter 12 discusses appraisal in more depth, particularly in relation to continuing professional development.

Coaching and Mentoring

Coaching and mentoring are key activities in medical education and career development. The purpose of both coaching and mentoring is to promote personal and professional development of the individuals and to help them take charge of their own development in order to achieve the results they desire.

Scenario 7.1

James is a third-year medical student allocated to a placement on a general medical ward (you first met James in Chapter 6). One of his learning outcomes for this placement is clerking patients and taking a history. He has to meet with his supervisor every week. Before his weekly meeting, he looks at his learning outcomes and reviews the work he has done to achieve these. This week, he has had an encounter with a patient on the ward that left him feeling worried and concerned. He felt that the pressure on him to extract key information from the patient in a short time span had made him act inappropriately and he wanted to discuss this with his supervisor. He writes about it in his reflective diary in preparation for the meeting. He sets out his reflection against the defined learning outcomes to help him as follows.

Learning Outcome

Obtain a patient's history and perform a physical examination in a logical, organized and thorough manner. Adapt to the urgency of the medical situation and the time available.

Reflective Entry

'It wasn't until I clerked my first patient, that I was better able to understand the consultant's behaviour. 'Just do a quick history and exam and present back to me in say 10 minutes?' I was asked by an F1. My patient was an elderly, mildly confused man. His story was jumbled and confused. I became impatient wanting to just extract the 'important' information from him. I tried to hurry him along mindful of the time, stopping him from telling me the 'softer' information. I was seeing the patient as a nuisance, someone that was disguising his own history from me – an obstacle to my efficiency. Almost immediately after the encounter, I began to feel terrible about how I had acted'.

During the meeting with his supervisor, they both agreed to focus on this issue. James provided more context in that he had seen how the consultant had not dealt fully with a patient's concern and had not wanted to emulate this behaviour. He felt he wanted to give more time to patients and their concerns but had felt the pressure to be 'quick' in his interactions with patients. James said he had found it helpful to write this down in the form of an imagined dialogue with one of his peers, Ravi (see Chapter 6).

They discussed where this pressure comes from, how it might be challenged and what strategies can be used in taking clinical histories, so as to extract key information whilst attending to a patient's concerns. Key learning resources were identified, and suggestions to look out for positive role models when interacting with patients. An action plan was agreed to be reviewed at the next meeting, which included working with the F1 and observing how she took histories.

The terms 'coaching' and 'mentoring' are sometimes used interchangeably (De Souza and Viney, 2014) and they may fulfil similar purposes, but there are differences. For example, the nature and the length of the relationship may be different between the two. Coaching may be a shorter-term relationship in which the coach specifically guides the individual in learning key aspects of practice that he or she may find difficult, such as learning how to communicate effectively with patients. Coaching is also helpful when an individual is at a 'career crossroads' and needs help in appraising options and making decisions. Mentoring is usually a longer-term relationship focused around personal and career development within a specific context or organization.

Coaching

Coaching emerged from and was inspired by sports coaching, with a focus on action. The coachee's own knowledge and experience together with that of the coach is used to improve the coachee's actions. Coaching was adopted by business and management and is linked with career development and performance. Some widely used models of coaching are the GROW (Whitmore, 2009) and the TGROW (Downey, 2003) models.

GROW is an acronym of goal, reality, obstacles and way forward. The 'goal' is the endpoint that the individual wants to achieve. It must be a SMART goal, that is, specific, measurable, attainable, realistic and time bound, so that the individual knows when it is attained. The 'reality' requires the current issues and the challenges to be stated before an assessment of how far away the individual is from the goal can be made. The 'obstacles' stopping the coachee attaining the goal need to be identified so that he or she can come up with different 'options', or ways to deal with them. The 'way forward' involves defining the necessary action steps required to achieve the goal, obtaining feedback from the coach and setting review dates.

In the TGROW model (Downey, 2003) the T stands for topic, to make sure that the context that affects the goals and actions is understood. The 'topic' item enables both the coach and the coachee to understand the 'context' of the issue to be addressed. This covers the wider environment that impacts on the specific issue to be addressed through coaching. It will reflect the level of importance the issue has within this wider area and the impact it may have on the coachee's long-term aspirations.

Coaching usually focuses on the behaviours and skills needed to function in a particular role. Whilst the coach is supportive, he or she should also challenge the learners' performance in order to encourage them to reflect and think critically about it. Donald Schön (whose work was discussed in Chapter 3) saw coaching as an essential element in learning the artistry of professional practice.

Table 7.1 Heron's six categories of interventions (Heron, 1986; Matthews, 2014; MindTools, 2016).

Who leads	Intervention	What you do or ask
The mentor or coach leads, more authoritative	Prescribing – where you would strongly suggest or require a specific action	• Give advice and guidance • Tell the other person how they should behave • Tell them what to do
	Informing – where you respond to a request, i.e. have been asked to find out something specific	• Give your view and experience • Explain the background and principles • Help the other person get a better understanding
	Confronting – where you may tell your mentee something that he or she may not want to hear	• Challenge the other person's thinking • Play back exactly what the person has said or done • Tell the person what you think is holding him or her back • Help the person avoid making the same mistake again
Mentee led, in that the mentor or coach is helping to facilitate the individual in finding solutions	Catalytic – where you would provide a stimulus for an action required as well as the motivation to be able to complete it	• Help the other person express feelings or fears • Empathize with the person
	Cathartic – where you would provide a safe place for your learner to discuss issues with you	• Ask questions to encourage fresh thinking • Encourage the other person to generate new options and solutions • Listen and summarize, and listen some more
	Supportive – where you would show and demonstrate support that may be required in response to your learner's needs	• Tell the other person you value him or her (his or her contribution, good intention or achievements) • Praise the person • Show the person he or she has your support and commitment

Mentoring

Mentoring may incorporate elements of coaching but has a different focus. The term 'mentor' originated in Greek mythology, where Mentor was the older counsellor and friend of Odysseus. It is typically associated with the provision of wise advice to less experienced individuals. In organizations, formal mentoring programmes allocate a more experienced individual to guide the less experienced in order for them to learn about the organization and reach their full potential. The mentor aims to help the mentee develop his or her career and associated personal and professional development, more broadly than simply developing specific behaviours and skills. This should be a confidential and supportive relationship in which there are shared values and trust between the individuals (Hodgson and Scanlon, 2013). The relationship can be formal or informal and usually develops over time, with less emphasis on structure than an appraisal or coaching relationship.

Coaching and mentoring are designed not necessarily to solve problems and issues for the learners but to help them see ways to solve them themselves. An important component of both of these activities is the ability for the coach or mentor to help the learner to be reflective in thinking forward and back on experiences, identifying what has been learned, what needs to be learned and what needs to be changed. Heron (1976) outlines six categories of interventions that the mentor can use with the mentee, split into two categories; see Table 7.1.

Summary

This chapter considers a range of face-to-face activities occurring in learning and clinical practice settings that incorporate reflection. Problem- and case-based learning were described, indicating how central the reflective process is to these learning activities. Activities that further support reflective learning, such as supervision, appraisal, mentoring and coaching, were discussed.

Reflection, Critical Thinking and Action Research

> Reflection and reflective practice are ways of developing and accessing knowledge about practice. In doing this, the reflective practitioner is engaged in research and critical inquiry as part of everyday practice. It is this research and critical inquiry aspect that will be examined in more detail in this chapter, through looking at the relationship between reflection, critical thinking and research. The chapter begins by considering reflection and knowledge generation, moves to critical thinking and outlines action research, concluding with some examples of action research in practice.

Connecting Reflection and Knowledge Generation

Reflection *in* or *on* practice serves several purposes. The one most discussed in this book so far is how reflecting on practice can help to identify the knowledge that was used in practice situations and any knowledge deficits that there may have been. By reflecting *on* action and analysing the incident in depth it is anticipated that some learning will occur.

As we saw in Chapter 3, reflection and reflective practice has a long history. However, Rolfe (2014) argues that the radical nature and roots of reflective practice may have been misunderstood and lost. He reconsiders the work of Donald Schön (1983) in arguing that it is reflection *in* action rather than reflection *on* action that is important. He reiterates that Schön's work was a critique of technical–rational knowledge and agrees that such knowledge is useful in solving 'tame' problems but has limitations in solving 'wicked' problems (Rittell and Webber, 1973, cited by Rolfe, 2014). Both tame and wicked problems are seen in clinical practice, but it is the wicked ones that expose the limitations of technical–rational knowledge. Take for example the Enhanced Recovery after Surgery Pathway (Kehlet, 1997). This sets out evidence-based guidelines for the management of the patient undergoing surgery through all stages of the peri-operative process. This pathway is largely based on technical–rational

Developing Reflective Practice: A guide for medical students, doctors and teachers, First Edition.
Andrew Grant, Judy McKimm and Fiona Murphy.
© 2017 John Wiley & Sons Ltd. Published 2017 by John Wiley & Sons Ltd.

knowledge derived from research and other forms of evidence. It is extremely useful in the management of surgical patients, but only, and this is Rolfe's point, if everything goes to plan. If the patient's progress through the peri-operative process is unproblematic it remains a *tame* problem. However, if the patient deviates from the pathway, perhaps through an unexpected anaesthetic event or bleed, then the problem becomes a *wicked* one. The anaesthetist or surgeon may have to rapidly reflect in action, mentally running through his or her repertoire of strategies gained not just from knowing the technical–rational evidence but drawing on his or her years of experience (Delany and Golding, 2014). The doctors have to theorize *in* action and experiment and test this theorizing *in* action to solve the problem. In this way, the practitioner is theorizing, hypothesizing and actively experimenting. This process and the knowledge gained from this process should also be a source of legitimate knowledge for clinical practice, which is as important as 'evidence-based' guidelines (Greenhalgh, Howick and Maskrey, 2014).

Rolfe (2014), in supporting Schön's ideas, argues that technical–rational knowledge, despite its limitations for professional practice, remains dominant. He further argues that the use (or possible misunderstanding) of reflective practice has only served to perpetuate this and has not really challenged the dominance of technical–rational knowledge in the evidence-based practice movement (Rolfe, 2014). Comer (2016) argues that Schön's writings can be interpreted in different ways, but Rolfe (2014) reminds us that being reflective should also incorporate critical thinking in order, if not to challenge the status quo, at least to be aware that it exists. From this perspective, practitioners themselves in the 'swampy lowlands' (Schön, 1983) are the researchers, theory builders and knowledge generators, not just the experts on the 'hard high ground' (Schön, 1983).

Connecting Reflection, Knowledge and Research through Critical Thinking

Part of the reflective practice movement has been linked to ideas around not just thinking but critical thinking. To take action we need to take a critical stance to really examine the underlying assumptions and beliefs that shape what we do and how we and others think. We need to understand how 'social structures' such as social class, gender and ethnicity shape and form the power relationships around individuals, and how this influences our everyday practice (Finlay, 2008; Morton-Cooper, 2000, p. 76). Reflection can help us to look at ourselves and the world around us, but we also need to be critical thinkers. Critical reflection is more likely to lead to change, not just at the individual level, but in wider transformative action through social action.

As discussed in Chapter 3, various definitions of critical thinking exist, and Brookfield (1987) suggests that there are four components (Figure 8.1). We will look at these components using an example described in Box 8.1.

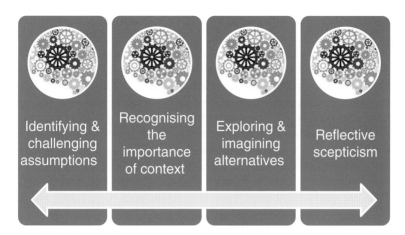

Figure 8.1 Components of critical thinking (after Brookfield, 1987).

Box 8.1 Exposure

I and three other medical students were invited to watch an ultrasound being performed by a senior radiologist as part of a teaching session. We were invited into the room prior to the patient, and the radiologist proceeded to explain the equipment he would be using to us. An auxiliary and nurse then brought in the patient; an elderly woman, who was blind and had difficulty standing. She was complaining of abdominal pain and required an ultrasound of her kidneys. The nurse and auxiliary helped the patient from her wheelchair and onto the bed with some difficulty. They then helped her to get comfortable, and exposed her stomach. During this time, which was considerable due to the patient's difficulty mobilising, the radiologist continued to explain the equipment and procedure to us without so much as acknowledging the patient's presence. He then proceeded to apply gel and place the ultrasound probe on the patient's abdomen whilst continuing to talk only to us, before eventually telling her he was scanning her kidneys.

The radiologist continued to scan patient's kidneys using some pressure, causing the patient to become visibly uncomfortable. However, the radiologist made no acknowledgement of this until much later, finally asking the patient "does that hurt?" in a nonchalant manner. He made no effort to make the patient more comfortable, and on conclusion of the procedure simply pronounced it "Finished!" before continuing his teaching. The patient was left to be helped into her wheelchair and wheeled out by the nursing staff.

The situation was obviously made worse by the patient's inability to see; she was brought into a room and exposed considerably in front of a group of persons she would not be able to identify, and at no point had our presence explained. The experience made some of my colleagues and the nursing staff visibly uncomfortable, and left me personally feel very angry about the patient's treatment.

1. Identifying and Challenging Assumptions

Sometimes facts, emotions and opinions can get tangled up together, which is why frameworks such as the one proposed by Gibbs (1988) consciously make the person identify what his or her feelings were around the event. It is also evident that individuals bring their own unique interpretations to events, as the same event can be experienced by different people, yet each might have a different interpretation. To help to recognize assumptions underpinning interpretations of events, Finlay (2008) and Bassot (2012) discuss Brookfield's (1998) four critical lenses. These were originally used in relation to teaching teachers, but are also useful in clinical practice. Brookfield argues that to be critically reflective 'we need to find some lenses that reflect back to us a stark and differently highlighted picture of who we are and what we do' (Brookfield, 1998, p. 197). These four critical lenses (modified for healthcare) (Figure 8.2) are

- our own autobiography
- our patients' and clients' eyes
- our colleagues' experience
- the theoretical literature.

Our Autobiography

As a learner or qualified practitioner, our previous experiences of being a learner and of health and healthcare shape how we view and interpret situations. It is therefore important to be aware of how earlier experiences might influence our view and responses to events. For example, if as a child you had

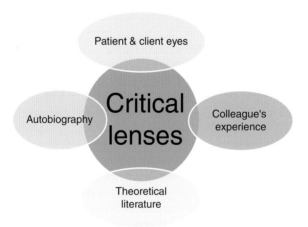

Figure 8.2 Four critical lenses (after Brookfield, 1998).

a poor experience at school or have felt humiliated by domineering teachers, you may be less likely to speak out in groups or on ward rounds. Brookfield makes the point that, whilst individual experiences are unique to that person, there may be similarities in others' experiences that we can connect with in helping us to understand our own experience. Group reflective processes can be helpful in enabling us to share our experiences and see how others view the world, and can help to challenge assumptions.

Our Patients' and Clients' Eyes

Brookfield, referring to teacher education, identified that it is the view through the learners' eyes that is of significance. In healthcare, we need to try to see through the patients' and clients' eyes to try to understand how our actions might be seen by those we are caring for. Part of a group or one-to-one reflective process is to help the individual see his or her actions through the eyes of the patient. What we consider as appropriate or routine actions might not be viewed that way at all by the person or family receiving our actions and behaviour. It is easy to forget that, for many patients, coming to hospital, physical examination and tests are frightening. Like healthcare workers, patients have their own autobiography, which also shapes their interpretation and response to events. For example, an older person coming into a hospital that used to be a workhouse or mental asylum will feel very different from you: he or she may see it as somewhere people don't come out from, whereas for you it is 'just' your workplace. Listening to and reflecting on people's stories, fears and concerns helps you to develop deeper understanding and connections.

Our Colleagues' Experiences

The critical lens theme continues in imagining our actions when seen by colleagues. In a group reflective session, the colleagues might be fellow students, who may offer a different way of seeing, interpreting and responding to the event that has happened. If this is constructive it can be very helpful to have different interpretations and responses to the situation. Brookfield suggests that through describing individual experiences, common problems and issues can be identified, as well as points of difference. What the group can do is to suggest a repertoire of explanations and strategies to help deal with issues. In the example in Box 8.1, the radiologist's perspective was not explored but might have offered a different perspective on the incident.

Theoretical Literature

Part of the reflective process is to identify gaps in knowledge, so it is necessary to consider some of the theories and knowledge taught in healthcare programmes. This theoretical literature can expand thinking and knowledge in different directions as well as helping to consolidate what is already known.

These four 'critical lenses' are therefore useful to help to identify and challenge assumptions and viewpoints, enabling situations to be seen in a different way.

2. Recognizing the Importance of Context

The second component of critical thinking is recognizing the importance of context. Brookfield sees this as a way of lifting our heads up from examining just ourselves to looking at the wider context. For example, context can relate to the culture of a setting in which there are unwritten rules as to expected behaviour. In Box 8.1, an uncomfortable situation is described in which the nurses and medical students did not say anything despite their discomfort. These types of question are often concerned with issues of power and its use (or abuse) in healthcare. Taylor (2010) suggests that we need to use 'emancipatory reflection' to examine power structures. Through such reflection, the individual becomes aware of the power relations within any interaction, starts to question these power relations and potentially has the ability to transform these relations to emancipate him- or herself and others. Taylor identifies four stages in emancipatory reflection: constructing, deconstructing, confronting and reconstructing.

Constructing

This is describing as richly as possible a situation where the individual might have felt he or she did not make a difference because there was an imbalance in power relations. In Box 8.1, the individual describes the situation clearly and identifies feelings of disquiet and unease as to what happened.

Deconstructing

From the description and feelings identified, Taylor suggests looking for and being aware of the power relations that may be very clearly evident in the situation or hidden from view. We asked earlier why the medical students or nurses did not intervene. The answer might lie in the power relations involved in this situation, as the radiologist is perceived to have more power than the other individuals. Both Taylor and Brookfield recommend standing outside ourselves and trying to see the incident as an interested observer might to begin to make sense of the situation.

Confronting

Having become aware of the power relations in the situation, Taylor recommends asking some key questions to further explore this (Taylor, 2010, p. 152, adapted from Smyth, 1996).

- Where do the ideas I embody come from historically?

- How did I come to appropriate them?
- Why do I continue to endorse them?
- Whose interests do they serve?
- What power relations are involved?
- How do these influence my relationships with the people in my care?
- What cultural, economic, historical, social and/or personal constraints are operating in this practice story?

To answer some of these questions, an interested observer with recourse to the theoretical literature (Brookfield, 1987) might draw on ideas from the history of medicine, the development of medicine as a profession, the socialization or enculturation processes of medical students within medical education, the transmission of norms and values through these processes, the relationship and power dynamics with other occupations such as nursing, the power relations within the doctor–patient relationship, and how patients move into the 'sick role' and become *medicalized*. This kind of analysis takes individuals beyond themselves to recognition of the wider cultural, historical and social factors that have shaped them and shaped the context for this experience.

Reconstructing

Given this new-found awareness, Taylor argues that the next step must be to transform and change, and she asks 'in the light of what I have discovered, how might I work differently?' (Taylor, 2010, p. 153). This need for change can be seen in the models of reflection discussed in Chapter 4. Taylor acknowledges how difficult this kind of transformative change is for individuals and how collective action might be a strategy to adopt. In the incident outlined in Box 8.1, it was obviously difficult for the individuals to behave as they felt would be more appropriate, but understanding the power relations gives some insight as to why this might be the case.

3. Exploring and Imagining Alternatives

Having identified and challenged assumptions and recognized the importance of context, the third component of critical thinking is to use our imagination and creativity to think of alternative courses of action (Brookfield, 1987). The critical lenses of the patients' and clients' eyes and our colleagues' experiences are particularly useful in helping us to understand that not everyone will share our perception and interpretation of events. These different perspectives might suggest different courses of action.

4. Reflective Scepticism

Brookfield's final component of critical thinking is 'reflective scepticism'. Although we may not agree with the perspectives generated from the critical reflective process, we need to evaluate the perspectives and arguments presented to draw conclusions. When experiences and assumptions are examined through these different lenses a more in-depth and broader perspective on the experience is gained.

Action Research: Connecting Reflection, Knowledge and Critical Thinking

Critical thinking in this way helps to connect individual experiences with the wider social context. Individual practitioners may berate themselves over their perceived inability to give good patient care. However, if they stepped back from their own experience to consider the wider context they would see that, for example, economic systems, government policies, politics and resource allocation all potentially shape the care that can be provided by any one individual. This kind of social and political analysis is essential to bring about social action and is an important output from the reflective process.

Social action is linked to the research process through action research. Action research is defined by Greenwood and Levin (2007, p. 1) as 'a set of collaborative ways of conducting social research which satisfies scientific requirements and brings about social change'. Action research comprises three key elements: action, research and participation. Action research is seen as different from other ways of doing research (for example observational or experimental studies) in that it moves beyond simply studying the situation to trying to change it. Problems are identified; solutions are found and then implemented and evaluated as part of the action research cycle. Action research can be defined as practical, knowledge generating or emancipatory (Newton and Burgess, 2008). Working with participants as equals in bringing about change and generating knowledge about their world also leads to empowerment (Huang, 2010). What further distinguishes action research from other forms of research is the active participation by all stakeholders in the research process and the acknowledgement of the researcher as a key stakeholder. Action research is 'self consciously collaborative and democratic to generate knowledge and design action with trained "experts" and local stakeholders working together doing with rather than doing for' (Greenwood and Levin, 2007, p. 1). This kind of research approach lends itself readily to public and patient involvement initiatives (e.g. INVOLVE, 2009) in which the voice of the patient and service user is evident throughout the whole research process. Action research may also emphasize collaboration to produce knowledge (Bergold and Thomas, 2012) as well as action to change practice.

Figure 8.3 provides an overview of the research process, which can be applied to any type of research. However, in action research all these stages are participatory. The first stage of identifying a problem or area of interest is mutually and collaboratively arrived at. All stakeholders – patients, learners, administrators and healthcare professionals – work together collaboratively to identify the issues that are of concern to all of them. This can be a powerful process, in which no one stakeholder is seen to be more expert than the others. Rather, all bring different levels of expertise to the whole process and this expertise is used at different times in the process. All participants' contributions are taken seriously, with the diversity of knowledge and experiences being seen as an opportunity (Greenwood and Levin, 2007), as stakeholder insights into everyday practice are a crucial component of the process. The second stage of the research process therefore draws on more than just the literature in that the experience of the stakeholders also forms an important part of the 'evidence' that shapes the development of the research question, aims or hypotheses (the third stage).

The fourth stage of the research process is selecting the research approach, in this case action research. Action research has its origins in the work of Kurt Lewin (1946), a social psychologist interested in the process of change in industrial organizations. The later work of Paulo Freire (1970) in giving voice to oppressed minorities was also influential. This combination of influences results in a commitment to do research *with* people as participants and stakeholders

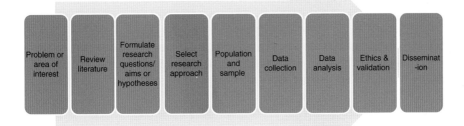

Figure 8.3 The research process.

rather than *on* people as subjects (Greenwood and Levin, 2007; Herr and Anderson, 2005). As indicated earlier, action research is an umbrella term (Herr and Anderson, 2005), which, although it covers a diversity of approaches, usually contains the three elements of action, research and participation, although a different emphasis may be placed on any of these components. Examples of different types of action research are participatory action research (Freire, 1970), educational action research (Carr and Kemmis, 1986), action science (Argyris, Putnam and Smith, 1985), 'new paradigm research' (Reason and Rowan, 1981), appreciative inquiry (Cooperrider and Whitney, 2005) and cooperative enquiry (Heron, 1996).

Regardless of the approach, action research is characterized by stages and cycles of action in which the ability to critically reflect is crucial (COBE, 2005, p. 5).

The problem or issue to be solved is identified, and possible solutions and interventions are also identified, implemented and then evaluated. Hence, in the fifth stage of the research process, the population and sample are carefully selected as to how they will inform each part of the action research cycle. More conventional understandings of purposive and nonpurposive sampling strategies may not be as relevant or applicable in this approach.

In terms of methods (the sixth stage of the research process), action research is pragmatic in that it draws on both qualitative and quantitative methods and thus may combine different types of method. Surveys, interviews, analysis of large data sets, experiments, blogs – whatever will work to implement and evaluate the solution to the identified problem or issue – will be used. This then affects the data analytical processes in the seventh stage of the research process.

The eighth step of the research process is ethics and validation. As with any research there are ethical considerations, and part of the action research process is to be aware of these and to be able to act in an ethical manner in the conduct of research. This type of participatory research can raise many complex ethical issues, for example potential tension between academic researchers and practitioners (Bergold and Thomas, 2012). Thus formal ethical approval is required once the design process is complete and before any research is carried out.

Proponents of action research argue that the process is rigorous; furthermore, it is valid in being action oriented in bringing about and sustaining change (Herr and Anderson, 2005, p. 49). A 'quality' action research project is characterized by how fully the participants are engaged in the process (Huang, 2010). Greenwood and Levin (2007, p. 3) further argue that the components of participation and action with research lead to 'a more just, sustainable, or satisfying situation for the stakeholders'. This is because it is designed to solve their problems, with the actions identified to solve the problems being owned by them, all of which contributes to the validity and rigour of the action-research approach.

The final stage of the research process is dissemination. The more conventional forms of dissemination such as producing papers for publication and conference presentations will still occur, with all stakeholders named as co-authors. There may be other less conventional forms of dissemination such as parties, social events and exhibitions. The difference here is to move away from the sole use of the academic third person to allow all participants' and stakeholders' voices to be heard.

Action research then can help practitioners critically reflect on and examine their work practices and interactions, and arrive at some kind of consensus on what kinds of service should be provided and why they need to be provided in a particular way (Morton-Cooper, 2000). In summary, action research is practitioner generated and workplace oriented. It starts with a shared problem and aims to improve practice, in which examining assumptions and challenging them is key. The research approach can be cyclical and flexible and there may be no final definitive answers at the end of the process (Morton-Cooper, 2000).

Examples of Action Research

Table 8.1 provides two examples of research projects that illustrate aspects of the action research process and types. In presenting these summaries, the framework of 'background', 'aim', 'approach', 'actions' and 'what happened?' as suggested by Huang (2010) is used.

Table 8.1 Examples of 'action research' projects.

Title	O'Sullivan, G., Hocking, C. and Spence, D. (2014) Action research: Changing history for people living with dementia in New Zealand. *Action Research*, **12** (1), 19–35.	Mendenhall, T.J. and Doherty, W.J. (2007) Partners in diabetes. Action research in a primary care setting. *Action Research* **5** (4), 378–406.
Background	Dementia services in New Zealand need to engage with people who have dementia and their families to provide support for a normal life for as long as possible.	Diabetes a growing problem. Single, expert-led conventional educational and psychosocial interventions are not sustainable. Need programmes that promote active participation of professionals and lay people.
Aim	Explore and uncover the support needs of people living with dementia.	Examining the processes within a Partnership in Diabetes project as an example of Citizens Health Care.
Approach	Action research underpinned by critical hermeneutics.	Participatory research.

(Continued)

Table 8.1 (Continued)

Actions	Regular meetings with 11 participants and their caregivers in the participants' own homes. Conversations were recorded and field notes taken of the participants' physical state and level of engagement. Participants were asked what topics they wanted to discuss. Followup of two focus groups with the participants to discuss the findings. Cycles of observation, reflection and action.	Qualitative analysis of the meeting notes (49 meetings over 3 years) of a Partners in Diabetes project group. Key informant interviews (4 professionals, 6 support partners – patients and spouses).
What happened	People with dementia are marginalized and stigmatized. There is a need for greater awareness of living with dementia and the inadequacy of service provision. The authors detail the actions that were taken which were around education, raising awareness and influencing policy decisions in New Zealand.	11 major themes identified, among them that healthcare providers and patients need to learn a different way of working. Providers and patients adopted leadership roles in the programme and identified training needs. The partner support role is very varied and they were key stakeholders. Challenges in the partnership process were identified.

Summary

This chapter has connected the different elements of reflection, knowledge, critical thinking and research. Reflection is about thinking. This thinking can be developed into critical thinking, in which individuals must critically examine their own interpretations and assumptions of their experiences. Critical thinking helps us to move beyond the individual experience to examining the wider context and the forces that impact on and shape individual action. Awareness of social issues leads to social action, and this is translated through action research, which has as core components the ideas of participation and action.

Part III

Facilitating Reflection

9

Teaching and Supporting Reflection

This chapter is written principally for teachers in medical (and health professions') education. It aims to help them support their learners when they use various reflective-learning techniques. It begins with techniques used to help learners get started with and get the most out of reflective learning. The chapter finishes with a discussion of how to integrate reflection into learning in a programme without the educational benefits being overshadowed by the need to assess reflective work.

If you are using (or are going to introduce) reflective learning with your learners, then you need to have a very clear idea of what the aims, goals and learning outcomes are: in other words, what is the specific purpose (or purposes) of reflective learning in your programme? It is a good idea at this stage to separate in your mind what learning needs to be acquired in relation to the subject matter and what learners need to demonstrate to prove that they have acquired reflective-learning skills as a way of being prepared for the lifelong learning involved in a medical or health professional career. Your learners will be happier if you can clarify what learning is required and to what level. Although this is true for any learning unit, what is different here is that you are asking learners to develop proficiency as reflective learners as well as achieving content learning outcomes. Learners who are uncertain of what is required from them may well respond with poor engagement and negative ideas towards the programme as a whole.

When introducing reflective learning to your learners for the first time, or introducing an unfamiliar reflective-learning task, you should expect some resistance and cynicism. Your task will be much easier if you are clear, in your own mind at least, about the reasons why you are using reflection and what you think your learners will gain. This means being sure of yourself without being patronizing or taking a 'we know best' approach, being assertive without being

Developing Reflective Practice: A guide for medical students, doctors and teachers, First Edition.
Andrew Grant, Judy McKimm and Fiona Murphy.
© 2017 John Wiley & Sons Ltd. Published 2017 by John Wiley & Sons Ltd.

defensive or dismissive: if it is important enough to be included in your pro-gramme, then it needs to be portrayed as meaningful and helpful for future practice. The suggestion is that by having the rationale for what you are intro-ducing and the supporting evidence clearly in your mind, your job in introduc-ing it to your learners will go much more smoothly. We often find that asking more senior learners who value reflection to talk to students is helpful, as they can relate it directly to clinical practice and explain the benefits.

The key questions that need to be addressed in order to be able to develop effective and meaningful reflective learning are given in Box 9.1 and explored further throughout the chapter.

Aims, Goals and Purpose

It is worth helping learners to keep in mind the goal of learning activities, which should be closely linked to any required output, such as a reflective diary, portfolio or essay (see Scenario 9.1). However, it is very easy for learners to focus on the output (and getting the assignment or module successfully completed and signed off). For the rest of this chapter our principal focus is going to be on helping your learners to achieve the best possible long-term learning outcomes as a return on the time they invest in reflective learning.

Box 9.1 Clarifying aims and learning outcomes: asking the right questions

1) What are the overall aims of the programme?
2) What strategies will be used to ensure that learners know what is expected of them and how they will receive feedback?
3) Are the learning outcomes that will need to be achieved in order to reach these goals clearly stated using appropriate language and written in a SMART format (see Box 10.3)?
4) How will introducing reflection enhance your learners' learning?
5) How will your learners choose what they reflect on?
6) How will your learners capture these events?
7) How much structure will you want your learners' reflections to have?
8) How will your learners record their reflections?
9) Will learners share their reflections with anybody? If so
   a) who?
   b) what ground rules will make this sharing feel safe?
10) How will you know if reflective learning has taken place?
11) What strategies will be used to discourage learners from writing what they think the tutor wants to read or will gain them maximum marks?

Scenario 9.1 Learning from practice

Let's imagine, for example, that as part of an attachment in surgery you ask your learners to keep a reflective portfolio. The goal is to enable them to have the best learning experience during this attachment and to go away having achieved the best possible development of knowledge and skills in surgery (and more generically as a future doctor). They need to develop their metacognitive skills as they reflect on their learning (see Chapter 2). The final output, the portfolio, is just that: a physical (or electronic) record of reflective-learning activity during the attachment. If learners complete the placement having produced an impressive-looking portfolio, but have not developed their learning, then the placement, for them, has not been successful. By contrast, if the learner has a rich and varied learning experience but does not submit an adequate portfolio, their teachers have no idea what, if any, learning activity has taken place and will not be able to confirm that an adequate record of learning has been completed.

Most of us are, to some extent, strategic learners. That is to say, we learn according to the requirements made by programmes and courses or modules (for example, concentrating on what is expected to come up in the examination, or writing a learning journal in a way that is most likely to be deemed satisfactory). It is always tempting to work out what minimum effort will satisfy the examiners that the task has been completed satisfactorily. This is a healthy survival technique, and an element of it is always going to be present as we cannot learn everything. However, it is always worth challenging this approach and helping learners to carry out learning tasks so that they get the best learning experience rather than just progressing through the programme. Activity focussed on long-term learning may require little or no extra effort but will require thought at the planning stage. It is always a good idea to ask some learners to give you their thoughts and comments when planning reflective (and indeed any other) learning activities. They may help you see a reflective-learning activity from their strategic perspective rather than from your own focus, which is the intended learning. They may be able to point out to you how a strategic learner could successfully complete a reflective-learning task without achieving any of the true intended learning outcomes. We discuss this further in Chapter 10.

Supporting Learners to Get Started as Reflective Learners

When learners are first required to use reflection as part of their learning, it is to be expected that many will struggle with this new and (probably) unfamiliar mode of learning (Krause, 1996). Indeed it is suggested that overcoming this initial reluctance helps to develop the eventual satisfaction that is achieved (Krause, 1996). Many learners will also want to 'get it right' from the outset rather than learn through experience and reflection – which is the whole point of reflection after all (Grant, Berlin and Freeman, 2003)!

The simple set of guidelines in Box 9.2 was developed to help groups of medical learners to use a reflective-learning portfolio on placement in general practice (Pink, Cadbury and Stanton, 2008). When first introduced to reflective learning, many learners are reluctant to participate and may be resistant. In many cases this is because they have unrealistic ideas of what they are going to be asked to do. Some learners equate reflective learning with having to articulate their innermost thoughts and beliefs in front of teachers and peers. Therefore, some time explaining exactly what you do and do not expect your learners to do together in order to manage expectations is well spent. As well as management of expectations, Pink and colleagues found that giving learners an easy reflective-learning task to carry out initially, along with, if possible, some easy, early learning gains, can give learners a positive early experience. After the first task or session, an early debrief helps to reassure learners that they have understood the tasks asked of them, identify some positive aspects of the task and address any concerns that arise.

Selecting the Right Method of Reflective Learning

Although it is essential to select a reflective-learning method where the outcomes are well defined and the learners know what they have to do, it is also important to ask whether the chosen method is one that is compatible with

---

Box 9.2 Helping learners get started with reflection (Pink, Cadbury and Stanton, 2008)

The general principles of getting learners started with reflective learning apply to any new activity, but attention to the following items should get learners started quickly and with obvious early benefits:

- start with a relatively simple learning task, such as talking aloud with a peer;
- give learners enough information so that they are clear what they have to do;
- where possible give information just in time;
- address learners' concerns and be clear what you are *not* asking them to do (they may be worried that you will ask them to expose their innermost thoughts and feelings when you will not);
- debrief learners promptly after their first cycle of reflective learning.

Scenario 9.2 Reflection – an introductory morning

Graduate-entry medical students at Swansea University Medical School spend a significant amount of clinical placement time on *clinical apprenticeships*. These placements are where they learn the generic skills required of qualified doctors and take place in a wide variety of healthcare settings. At the end of these apprenticeships, students write an unstructured reflection, which may cover any aspect of their learning and development on the apprenticeship. Before writing the first reflective entry, the first-year students spend a morning being introduced to reflective practice and reflective writing.

Working in small groups with a facilitator, students are asked to write a reflection based on a recent experience, preferably from one of their early clinical placements. They then share their reflection, initially with one other student and then with a small group. Following this, the students are helped to recognize what has been added to the initial experience by reflecting on it. The students then, immediately, use the same framework to examine the cycle of reflective learning they have just carried out. Feedback suggests that students find that this double cycle of reflection on a learning experience followed by 'reflection on reflection' helps them to clarify what is required in their reflective commentaries and what they might expect to gain.

---

learners' prior experience and one where learners can see how reflection will enable them to achieve what they think they need to achieve (Sandars, 2008; Grant *et al.*, 2006).

Let us revisit the questions from Box 9.1, adding further detail as required.

1) *What are the overall aims of the programme?* In other words, what are you trying to achieve with your learners? For example, safe, competent, knowledgeable, reflective, caring and compassionate doctors.

2) *Are the learning outcomes that will need to be achieved in order to reach these aims clearly stated, using appropriate language, and written in a SMART format?*

> Specific – the outcome must be precise and as unambiguous as possible.
> Measurable – the outcome must be able to be measured in some way, usually through assessment (see Chapter 10).
> Achievable – for the stage of education or training and ability of the learners.
> Realistic – achievable with a reasonable amount of effort and appropriate to the context and practice.
> Time bound – the outcome must be able to be achieved within a specified timeframe.

To what level do you want your learners to achieve these learning outcomes? Using a hierarchical structure of learning levels with appropriate verbs for each level, such as 'Bloom's taxonomy' (Anderson, Krathwohl and Bloom, 2001), will help you to set this out clearly. Whilst this is a fairly mechanistic method, it is useful to conceptualize the learning outcomes in terms of knowledge and understanding, practical or transferable skills and (professional) behaviours. This then helps you select the most relevant teaching and learning methods and assessment activities.

These first two questions are fairly generic and will help you clarify your ideas when you start to plan any programme or course. You are more likely to achieve your goals if you define them clearly and refer to them regularly. Once the planning process gets under way it is extremely easy to be distracted by the learning strategies, the resources required and the assessments.

3) *What strategy(ies) will be used to ensure that learners know what is expected of them and how they will receive feedback?*
This requires a combination of clarity of learning outcomes (see Question 2) and time invested in introducing learners to reflective learning, clarifying its purpose and allaying any misunderstandings.

4) *How will introducing reflection add to your learners' learning?*
This is the single most important question. Your learners are much more likely to benefit in the way you intend if you are clear what you are setting out to achieve using reflection. In your introduction of reflective learning, are you more keen that your learners will finish the course having gained competence in reflective learning or do you want them to have achieved learning outcomes having used reflective methods? It is very likely that you will want them to have achieved both outcomes to some degree, in which case ask yourself which activity is the more important in terms of percentage of importance.

5) *How will your learners choose what they reflect on?*
Reflective learning will be unlikely to occur if you do not guide your learners in how to identify material on which to reflect. At the outset this will not seem obvious or natural to your learners, and if you do not help them they may feel uncomfortable and out of their depth. Some introductory exercises will help, but most importantly you need to empower your learners and to give them confidence that the material *they* choose is what is important. Conversely, the learners need to get the message clearly that they should never choose something to reflect on purely because they think it will gain favour with their teacher or a satisfactory grade.

6) *How will your learners capture the events they reflect on?*
In many situations, learners will not be able to write a reflective account of an event as soon as it happens. A medical student on a ward round who is

particularly impressed by the way a consultant breaks bad news to a patient and what they might learn for their own practice in the future may be able to write brief notes in a notebook or dictate a voice message on their mobile phone as an aide memoire. They could then reflect on this in depth later when they have time (see Chapter 7 for more ideas on reflective activities). Learners should be encouraged to develop a method of capture of events on which to reflect that suits them and their way of learning. Different methods of reflection involve processing information in different ways. Learners should be encouraged to find methods of representing events that make it easy for them to reflect. If using a visual format such as a drawing or mind map works for them, they should be encouraged to represent their reflection in this way. Many of your learners will carry smart phones and these make capture either by short written notes or by a brief audio recording very easy. The most important thing to get across in relation to capture is the concept of 'That's an interesting/stimulating/challenging event. I'd like to reflect on that when I have time.'

7) *How much structure will you want your learners' reflections to have?*
This takes us back to Question 1. If you want your learners to use reflection in a highly cognitive way, using reflection as a metacognitive tool to identify what they know and where the gaps are in their knowledge, then you might utilize fairly prescriptive reflective templates that lead the learner through the points of a reflective-learning cycle such as the ones by Kolb or Gibbs (see Chapter 4). You can adapt these reflective-learning cycles for specific learning conditions or environments. For example, final-year medical students have a particular need to be ready for work as first-year foundation doctors (interns) when they graduate, and, more specifically, to be able to assess acutely ill patients and act appropriately (including calling for more experienced help where necessary). Questions can be added to the usual reflective template to ask, specifically, if and how the learner gathered appropriate information about the patient's current medical state, what action they planned to take, their evaluation of their performance, what they had learned and what they would do differently in a similar situation in future. Remember that highly unstructured or free-form reflections are difficult to mark summatively with consistency.

8) *How will your learners record their reflections?*
Learners are more likely to respond favourably, and therefore benefit educationally, if completing their reflective learning is an easy and satisfying process. If at all possible, use an online format. This has the advantage of being accessible from any computer, tablet or smart phone and will give the learner a better record of their reflection, which they can refer back to at a later stage.
It is vital that learners can easily look back at their reflective entries over time to see how their knowledge and reflective-learning skills have developed.

9) *Will your learners share their reflections with others?*
Reflection is not just about writing a personal reflective journal or diary. Although the act of writing and reflecting on an event has the effect of getting a learner to process the information relating to that event, this need not be the only processing that happens. Through working regularly in a small group, learners can share their reflections. By doing this they can learn from the events their peers have reflected on as well as their own. These groups may need to be facilitated to start with, but once learners have experienced the benefit of a reflective-learning group they can lead the group themselves, appointing one of their number to act as chair (see Box 9.3). If this is not possible, perhaps because learners are widely spaced on clinical placements, they can give their peers access to their online reflections and share comments and reactions through an asynchronous chat room or discussion board. Learners might also submit their reflections to a tutor, who can give online comments. If the same tutor offers this over a period of time, then a Socratic dialogue may develop.

10) *Will learners' reflective learning be assessed?*
In order to answer this question, you will need to decide how much it matters whether your learners acquire the ability to learn using reflection. If, on graduation, they are going out into the clinical workplace where patients' presentations are complex and knowledge goes out of date very quickly it *is* essential. If it is an essential skill then, like any other learning outcome, your learners (and you) will need evidence that this skill has been acquired, and to the required level. This cannot be achieved unless the skill and required level have been clearly defined.

11) *How will you know if reflective learning has taken place?*
In order for your learners to gain the maximum learning benefit from reflection it is imperative to get this right. When you think about assessment go back to Question 2. What are the outcomes you want from the course? What evidence will show you that this has been achieved? Go back to your SMART learning outcomes and be clear whether you are looking for evidence of subject learning, improved proficiency in reflective learning (and/or writing) or a combination of the two. Make sure that all these outcomes are written in a form that is clear to learners and assessors.

12) *What strategies will be used to discourage learners from writing what they think the teacher wants to read or they think will gain them good marks?*
It is important to minimize the effect that assessment may have on metacognitive, intrinsically motivated learning. It is easy for learners to fix on assessment requirements while their teachers focus on the process of learning. Chapter 10 discusses assessment in more depth. Having to submit reflective work for assessment causes a conflict for many learners. Where learners are

writing very personal reflections they are justified in wanting to know exactly the criteria on which their work is going to be marked. Anyone asking a group of learners to reflect and to submit their reflective work should expect their learners to have concerns like these and should address them.

Using Learning Technologies to Enable Reflection

As we have discussed previously, learning technologies, particularly digital media, have opened up a range of opportunities for learners to engage in reflective activities that were not available before. Here we discuss some of the options available through e-learning and mobile learning.

E-learning has many different definitions, but essentially is learning using electronic means (including laptops and PCs), whereas mobile (or m-) learning is that specifically using mobile devices such as smart phones and tablets. Most universities and other organizations make use of a virtual learning environment (VLE) such as Blackboard™ or Moodle™. These usually have an inbuilt journal or portfolio function, which can be helpful for your learners to use to make reflective entries from any PC, tablet or smart phone. However, if this is all an online portfolio enables them to do over and above a paper-based format, it is being used as an online repository for reflective writings, in other words, an administrative tool. E-learning methods are therefore most appropriately used to add value to the reflective-learning process.

Value may be added by

- speeding up communication and feedback between learner and tutor, enabling rapid dialogue,
- sharing of reflective entries between groups of learners, with or without the input of a facilitator (this may be of particular value when groups of learners are dispersed, e.g. on clinical placements) or
- giving learners ready access to examples of previous learners' reflective work.

Take time to find out what is already available within your institution and whether this would require adaptation for your purposes. Speak to colleagues who already use the platform so that you are aware of the strengths and weaknesses and can learn from their experience. There are specific journal/reflection platforms (e.g. PebblePad™), which may be available via your institution or by taking out a subscription just for your learners. Bespoke reflective journals and/ or portfolios can be constructed if no readily available package will carry out the tasks you want, but this will almost certainly involve much expenditure of time and effort. Additionally, if you decide to develop a bespoke system will need commitment from your IT department not only to support the development of your online platform but also to provide ongoing support and development once it is in use. Bear in mind also that commercially available packages are, in general, easier to troubleshoot than bespoke ones (where in the worst case only the person who wrote the programme can fix any bugs).

Many of the platforms used for VLEs also give accessibility through apps for mobile devices, although functionality is often more limited or impaired; for example, Blackboard offers Blackboard Mobile Learn, PebblePad offers Pebble Pocket, and the national e-portfolio used for UK doctors in training can be used on mobile devices. In addition, it is becoming more common for learners (and therefore their teachers) to make much more use of mobile devices in capturing reflections using inbuilt functions such as digital recording, videos and note taking. These functions have the advantages of convenience and accessibility in that learners can capture learning events as soon as possible after they occur, many learners already have a smart phone and they do not need to worry about accessing external sites through firewalls or other barriers. As with any learning medium, you will need to define clearly what you expect your learners will gain through the introduction of reflective-learning activities using mobile technologies and how you will measure whether this has taken place.

Peer Learning

Most people reading this chapter will have had the experience of working with a group of their peers, possibly on a shared project or preparing for an examination, and know what a mutually beneficial experience this can be. The mutual support of a group of peers is equally applicable to reflective learning. A regular reflective-learning group, with or without a facilitator, can help learners to establish reflective practice and to gain further benefit from both presenting their reflective-learning material to the group and hearing about their peers' experiences.

As with other reflective-learning experiences, learners need to be very clear what is expected of them and what they might expect to gain. To function safely peer groups will need to have clear, mutually agreed ground rules, which should, at least, include confidentiality and mutual respect between group members (see Box 9.3). The reflective-learning group can provide a forum for learners to discuss the encounters they have chosen to include in their journal or portfolio for reflection. Clearly it is helpful for the group member presenting the encounter to have questions and challenges from the different viewpoints of their peers. In time, members can begin to recognize the behaviour and learning patterns of their peers. They are then, with tact and sensitivity, able to challenge their peers and help them recognize these patterns.

Box 9.3 Reflective-learning groups

Each group should agree its own set of ground rules. The following possibilities should be discussed:

- confidentiality within the group is essential if learners are going to feel safe to discuss their reflections;
- respect should be shown to every member and their reflections, no reflection is *wrong, stupid* or *irrelevant*;
- the time allocation and process needs to be agreed between the group members;
- only one member should speak at any one time;
- acceptable and respectful ways to challenge other group members must be agreed.

The facilitator's role should be clarified:

- to make sure all group members get a chance to speak;
- not to approve or disapprove of learners' reflections;
- not to act as a therapist or counsellor to the group or to individual members.

In addition to receiving help with the encounters that they themselves have chosen to reflect on, by attending the peer group members have the opportunity to hear about the encounters raised by their peers, which may act as a beginning (encounter) for cycles of reflective learning. This may bring to their attention other areas where they need to advance their knowledge or may present different perceptions on areas they are already aware of as needing attention.

Reflection as Part of Developing Professional Identity

The assumption underlying much of this chapter is that reflection is used, in learning, at least to some extent to support learning from experience. Through metacognition, learners gain a better idea of what they know, what they need to know and how they will address the gaps in their learning that they identify for themselves. This is, indeed, a potent way in which reflection can make a difference to learning throughout the learner's life, but it is not the only way in which health professionals can support their learning and development through reflective practice. As well as acquiring knowledge and skills, learners in the health professions also develop an identity, that of a learner of medicine, nursing and so on, and eventually a practitioner. In the terminology of Jean Lave and Etienne Wenger's *Situated Learning* (Lave and Wenger, 1991), they are, with time, occupying a more central place in their chosen *communities of practice.* We discuss the development of professional identity through reflection in detail in Chapter 11, but it is useful here to think about possible topics that might be covered by learners reflecting on their personal identity: see Box 9.4. If you want to encourage reflection on emergence and development of professional identity, then questions that invite learners to explore these aspects can be introduced into written or other reflective activities.

The first part of this chapter concentrated on experiential learning, where the learner uses a structured approach to reflection on learning encounters. This form of reflection often (though not always) focuses primarily on the learners' knowledge, where they are stimulated to examine existing knowledge and to identify learning needs. Sometimes, however, the principal intended outcome of reflection is that the learners should become more aware of the professional identity they are developing as they progress through their education and training. This form of reflection is typically less structured than knowledge-based reflections and may involve learners examining their values and beliefs and the effect of their cultural background on these. It is even more important that learners are able to do this

---

Box 9.4 Reflecting on emerging professional identity

Areas that may be covered when reflecting on developing professional identity include

- recognition of personal values and beliefs;
- recognition of source of personal values and beliefs;
- reactions to issues involving severe illness, injury and death;
- reactions to certain groups of patients, e.g. older people, those with mental health issues or cancer, children, drug users, smokers;
- witnessed behaviour towards patients, families and other health workers that the learner would like to emulate;
- witnessed behaviour towards patients, families and other health workers that the learner would not like emulate;
- being (or not being) a legitimate member of the team and how that feels;
- issues of personal development;
- recognition of developing professional identity (thinking, talking, behaving like a doctor/nurse/dentist);
- reflection on development over time (e.g. reflecting on development and change since entering university and now);
- reactions and feelings at times of transition.

in a safe environment, where they are not judged and where they are free to write/speak in confidence. Some opportunity to discuss their developing identity after writing about it in a fairly unstructured way is important. Written feedback can provide this, but also face-to-face discussion with a tutor or a peer group can be supportive. Developing ground rules as suggested in Box 9.3 is very important when discussing such personal, deeply held issues. The ground rules may be worth revisiting after the group has met a few times to ensure that members are still happy and find out whether they wish to make any changes. The same rules in relation to having to submit reflection for assessment as discussed in Chapter 10 apply here too. Because reflection of this kind involves learners exploring their cultural backgrounds, attitudes and behaviours it is difficult for a teacher to say more than that this kind of reflection has been submitted satisfactorily. An assessor might well be able to give individual learners feedback that can help steer them and give them guidance as they reflect on their emerging development as professionals.

Evaluating Reflective Learning and Teaching

This chapter has focussed on ensuring that you and your learners are clear why you are introducing reflective learning into the curriculum or programme. In Chapter 10 we consider how best to assess whether your learners have achieved the learning outcomes you have defined. For a fully *aligned curriculum*, the learning outcomes, form(s) of assessment (measurement of what your learners have learned) and the evaluation of the effectiveness of your reflective-learning innovation should all be planned together. It is much more difficult to evaluate the long-term impact of an educational intervention such as reflection than to measure knowledge, as the ability to learn through reflection is a skill honed through practice, metareflection and feedback.

Evaluation measures the fitness of purpose of your reflective-learning intervention(s) within the whole programme using a range of metrics and methods. These include

- assessment results – formal measurements of your learners' reflective-learning skills;
- learners' feedback on enjoyment, satisfaction and impact on practice of reflective activities;
- learners' self-reports on how well they feel they are prepared to engage in reflective activities and whether and how this helps their practice;
- reports from employers, clinical teachers and others on the ability of your learners to reflect on practice and learn from situations and mistakes;
- qualitative methods such as focus groups and interviews with key stakeholders.

Summary

This chapter has discussed a range of individual, group learning and teaching activities that teachers might wish to utilize when introducing reflective-learning activities into a programme or developing them further. We have also noted the importance of ensuring alignment between learning outcomes, learning and teaching methods, and assessment, and noted some ways in which reflective activities might be evaluated.

10

Assessing Reflection

In this chapter we will explore if, when and how learners' reflective work should be assessed. We will also examine how having their reflections assessed might change the way learners approach reflective learning and may even undermine the intended learning outcomes.

When you introduce reflective learning into a programme you will need to decide how much it matters whether your learners acquire reflective-learning skills. There are a number of ways of embedding reflection into a programme without formally assessing this, although feedback of some form should always be given otherwise learners will simply approach this as a tick-box exercise (see Box 10.1 for an example).

Doctors in training have to submit a number of reflective pieces in their e-portfolio, which forms part of the annual assessment for progression to the next stage of training. They do not receive a grade or mark for the contents but they need to have completed their portfolio to a satisfactory standard. If they fail to do this over a period of time, this will put their registration at risk. Once fully qualified, practising doctors working in the UK have to submit an annual reflective portfolio for appraisal, which forms part of the General Medical Council's (GMC's) five-year revalidation cycle. The reflective-learning skills that students acquire at an early stage are essential for them to keep up to date in whichever branch of medicine they go into for the rest of their career, as evidence of reflection is required by the regulator (the GMC). For this reason, medical schools need robust evidence that learners have acquired reflective and metacognitive learning skills. Writeups of reflective-learning encounters (as described in Scenario 10.1) typically form part of the assessment that determines whether students have acquired these skills. Reflection then is a requirement for all medical students and practising doctors.

Developing Reflective Practice: A guide for medical students, doctors and teachers, First Edition.
Andrew Grant, Judy McKimm and Fiona Murphy.
© 2017 John Wiley & Sons Ltd. Published 2017 by John Wiley & Sons Ltd.

> **Scenario 10.1 Reflection in undergraduate medicine**
>
> Medical students, on final year clinical placements and student internships, write reflective accounts of learning encounters, which they submit for assessment. To guide them through Kolb's experiential learning cycle, they are asked to set out their reflective accounts under the following headings:
>
> - What happened?
> - What does this tell you about your current understanding?
> - What learning needs does this identify for you?
> - How have you addressed/will you address these learning needs?
> - How will you approach things differently in future as a result of this encounter?

What Are You Looking For in Reflective Assessment?

In order for learners to gain the maximum learning benefit from reflection it is imperative to get this right. When you think about assessment go back to Chapter 9, Box 9.1 and the questions that need to be asked about aims and learning outcomes. What evidence will you need to demonstrate that this has been achieved? In terms of SMART learning outcomes, you need to be clear whether you are looking for evidence of subject learning, evidence of proficiency in reflective learning or a combination of the two. In Scenario 10.1 the content of students' learning is important, but the primary outcome being measured is students' ability to identify and address their own learning needs through reflection (i.e. evidence of development of their reflective-learning skills). When you are designing assessments of reflection, ensure that the relevant outcomes are written in a form that is clear to learners, teachers and assessors and that the learning outcomes are fully aligned with strategies for teaching/learning and assessment (Biggs and Tang, 2011).

Marking Reflective Work – a Cause of Potential Conflict

Having to submit reflective work for assessment causes a conflict for many learners. Where they are writing very personal reflections they may be justified in wanting to know exactly the criteria on which their work is going to be marked and who is going to read what they write. Anybody assessing reflective work should expect learners to have such concerns and should address them without waiting for learners to raise them.

By including reflective learning in the skills we expect learners to acquire we are enabling them to leave university or postgraduate training with strategies that will, throughout their working lives, enable them to identify and address learning needs that emerge through experience. Bourner (2003) makes a helpful comparison between assessing reflective learning and assessing critical thinking. The latter has been an expectation in higher education for many years and can help us consider what exactly we want to assess in terms of written reflections. It is possible to devise a set of questions that help you to explore whether learners have interrogated the experiences on which their reflection is based in such a way as to question their current understanding, to recognize learning needs and to identify how they might take a different approach in future. Posing specific questions might be used to determine whether reflection has taken place, although you will need to determine appropriate questions for your particular learning context (Bourner, 2003). A set of questions such as these, which may be incorporated into a marking schedule (see Box 10.1 and Table 10.1 later), can make it easier for the assessor to determine whether true reflective learning has taken place rather than learners simply doing the minimum that will gain them a pass.

Effects of Making Reflective Learning Compulsory

If reflection is compulsory and assessed, then we should not be surprised if some learners will view it as yet another chore to be completed in the minimum time and with minimum effort. If submission for marking is a requirement, then some learners will write what they think will satisfy the marker and might fix on the marking schedule rather than on the benefits of reflective learning. If you decide that reflective learning does not have to be submitted for marking then some learners will not engage with it and will not then achieve the associated learning outcomes. There is, however, a middle way. If submission is compulsory but only for the assessors to ensure that the learners have engaged with the reflective task, accepting that different learners will approach

---

Box 10.1 Questions to determine whether reflective learning has taken place (Bourner, 2003)

1) What was it about the experience that engaged you?
2) What does this say about you and your values and beliefs?
3) How do you feel about what happened now?
4) What does this experience tell you about your strengths and weaknesses?
5) Are there other ways of viewing that experience?
6) What might you do differently?

Scenario 10.1 (continued)

When assessing the reflective accounts, markers identify any factual statements that are incorrect. However, their primary role is to ensure that learning through reflection on clinical encounters is taking place. Does student reflection follow the stages of the theoretical model (Kolb's experiential learning cycle in this case)?

Students are not allocated a mark. Markers measure whether students have met the learning outcomes and, if they have, a pass is awarded. Students who have not met the learning outcomes are given very clear feedback and are required to resubmit the assignment.

---

it in different ways, then learners are bound to participate but are not graded. They are instead only given individualized feedback. In the UK Foundation programme, doctors in training have to engage with reflective writing but it is ungraded, so an approach like this may work for some types of reflective writing.

Strategies to Discourage Students from Writing What They Think the Tutor Wants to Read or Will Gain Them Good Marks

You might think that this does not deserve a point all to itself but it is easy for learners to focus on assessment requirements to the detriment of wider learning, whilst teachers focus on the theoretical learning possibilities of a learning strategy. Our students have invested a major chunk of their lives in getting onto the medical programme and are now spending a great deal of effort and money completing it. We should not, therefore, be surprised that they focus on how to successfully complete the programme with the minimum number of hitches or delays. It is also easy to see that they might equate this to successfully negotiating the assessments. It behoves us, therefore, to look at an assessed reflective assignment from the student's point of view and ask whether students could make up events to reflect on (thereby missing the intended learning outcomes) and still pass. Do the learning outcomes give them scope to try to write what will gain them a 'satisfactory completion' or 'pass mark' while bypassing the intended outcomes?

Involve some students in the planning stage of your reflective-learning assignments (indeed all assignments). They will view your assessment from a very different perspective and spot where your intended learning outcomes can be partially or completely bypassed.

Table 10.1 Marking grid for a reflective-learning task based on the Kolb cycle using grading on an A–E rating scale.

Criterion/Grade	Excellent/A	Good/B	Pass/C	Bare pass/D	Fail/E
Narrative	clear, narrative goes beyond basic description of events	clear description of the event	adequate description	narrative of event but lacking clarity	no clear narrative
Reflection and identification of learning needs	perceptive evaluation of existing knowledge in light of event	some evaluation of existing knowledge	recognition of learning needs	some recognition of learning needs but with lack of clarity	no clear identification of learning needs; gives more narrative
Addressing learning needs	broad reading around the topic	reading that covers all reading needs	addresses some learning needs	some effort at addressing learning needs but evidence unclear	learning needs not addressed
Accommodation of new and prior learning	*explains how* new and existing learning are combined	evidence that new and existing learning have been matched up	evidence of some attempt at matching up new and existing learning	is able to describe new learning	no evidence
Engagement with the reflective task	goes beyond the basic requirement	clear evidence	sufficient engagement	some engagement	little or no engagement
Evidence of ability to learn using reflection	clear evidence with insight how it might be applied in future	evidence of learning using reflection	achieves some, but not all, aspects of the Kolb cycle	incomplete evidence	no evidence

Creating a Robust, Defensible Assessment for Your Students' Reflective Work

Assessment of reflective learning (like most forms of assessment) can be placed on a spectrum. At one end are pieces of reflective work that have to be submitted in order for them to be passed as satisfactorily completed (mandatory completion, but ungraded). At the other end of the spectrum is reflective work that is summatively marked and given a percentage, numerical or A–F grade. Between these lie pass–fail models. However, the differences between the marking strategies used might be less than you may think. All depend on a marker or assessor determining whether the work has reached a previously defined standard. The main difference between satisfactory completion and graded work is that for the latter the marker has to determine how well the submission meets defined criteria along a number of categories ranging from fail to excellent, whereas for satisfactory completion the marker makes a binary decision, against pass or fail criteria. See Table 10.1 for an example of graded criteria.

Depending on the work being assessed and its complexity, some reflective pieces make the assessors' job very difficult. If your reflective assessment is going to be defensible then your marking schedule needs to ensure a degree of reliability between assessors and between marks awarded by the same assessor at different times. One advantage of using just a pass–fail assessment is that there is one very clear-cut point which your assessors should be able to apply consistently. Table 10.2 sets out a simple pass–fail grid.

If you were using this in practice it would need to be developed further to make the criteria clear, and you would need to decide whether all or a majority of the criteria needed to be met for a pass. However, whichever assessment strategy you choose you will need

- SMART (see Chapter 9) learning outcomes that include the level of learning;

Table 10.2 Marking grid for a reflective-learning task based on the Kolb cycle using a pass–fail rating scale.

Pass	Fail
clear narrative description of event	poor or absent narrative
identifies learning needs	learning needs not identified
joins up new and existing understanding	no accommodation of new and existing learning
demonstrates appropriate investment of effort	little or no evidence of effort
evidence of ability to learn using reflection demonstrated through action points	no evidence of ability to learn using reflection

- an assessment grid that translates these learning outcomes into marks or pass–fail criteria;
- clear written instructions, training and debriefing for your assessors;
- analysis of the psychometric properties of your assessment that include, at least, a clear demonstration of its validity and demonstration of inter-rater and intra-rater reliability.

Where reflection is being used principally as a way of supporting learners developing professional identities, you may decide that the most important component of the assessment process is providing individualized written feedback to the student. See Scenario 10.2.

Ensuring Robust, Valid, Reliable Assessment

We have, already talked about situations where a learner's reflection might be deemed unsatisfactory and where this may have serious consequences. Depending on the regulations of the programme or organization, learners may have to remediate by completing outstanding reflections or writing additional pieces satisfactorily. In extreme cases, they may fail part or all of a programme. The main reasons learners fail are that the reflective writings are too brief, they fail to show evidence of sufficient engagement or (for qualified practitioners) they fail to submit an adequate annual portfolio for appraisal. As a decision to fail a reflective assessment is one that will affect the progression of learners or the future career and livelihood of a qualified practitioner, it has to be made in a robust and defensible way (Koole *et al.*, 2011).

Scenario 10.2 Marking unstructured reflective accounts

Scenario 10.1 describes how students at Swansea University Medical School carry out reflective writing at the end of clinical apprenticeships (placements). They are given complete freedom to choose the subject of their reflection so (unsurprisingly) work is submitted on a wide range of topics and they are encouraged to set this out in a variety of ways. The marker may deem that the submission is too brief or does not show evidence of a satisfactory level of engagement. In this case the students will be given the opportunity to resubmit that piece of reflective writing, with clear feedback from the marker telling them what they need to do in order to submit work that gets a pass second time. Students cannot progress to the next year of the programme until these pieces of reflective writing have all been submitted to a satisfactory level. A member of medical school faculty will give every student subjective, written feedback on his or her reflection, guiding students in their developing awareness of their emerging professional identity as well as their acquisition of clinical knowledge and skills.

The first step is to produce defined, transparent, unambiguous learning outcomes. These help you produce the criteria against which the assessment will be marked. Well-written learning outcomes help educators to develop clear assessment criteria; see Table 10.3, which is an example of requirements for a written reflective commentary produced as part of an academic programme. It is worth spending some time aligning learning outcomes and criteria, as this will help both learners and assessors.

Alongside this alignment, a robust, reliable system needs to be developed by which this measurement takes place. It is important to make sure that any assessment is valid. A valid assessment measures what it is supposed to measure. The example above sets out clear criteria that the learners must meet. As this assessment is part of an academic programme, the assessors want the learners to be able to apply models and theories to practice as well as to identify future professional development activities. If you were assessing something different, for example *reflection in action*, then the assessment would need to be practical, using observation and questioning techniques.

It is only ever worth measuring the reliability of an assessment when the questions about validity have been answered satisfactorily (otherwise you risk reliably measuring something that is not particularly useful). It is only going to be possible to determine what the assessment is intended to measure (its face validity) if we have defined this clearly. Only then can we ask whether our assessment does, indeed measure achievement of this aim. Once we have a valid assessment we should consider reliability. Reliable assessments are reproducible. A reliable assessment is where two or more assessors assessing the same piece of reflective work give the same grade, mark or outcome, when the same assessor at two points in time gives the same mark/outcome or when the assessment is repeated year on year with a similar mark distribution. If any of

Table 10.3 Learning outcomes mapped to assessment criteria.

Learning outcomes	Assessment criteria
learners will be able to apply a reflective model derived from the literature to structure their reflective commentary	a reflective model derived from the literature is used to structure the reflective commentary
learners will be able to support observations and reflections through citing appropriate literature, theories and concepts drawn from a range of sources from within and outside the course materials	observations and reflections are supported by citing appropriate literature, theories and concepts drawn from a range of sources from within and outside the course materials
learners will be able to demonstrate *reflection for action* through analysis of the situation described in the commentary	a section is included in the commentary that identifies clear actions in terms of future learning or practice

these are not the case, we have an unreliable assessment on which we should not be making high-stakes' decisions. Train your assessors, and ask them to mark examples (for example, asking them all to mark the same example as a training exercise) and then to discuss with each other the marks they have allocated. This will help them to develop a shared perception of the purpose of the assessment and to clarify how to apply the marking schedule. This, in turn, will enable them to mark consistently and reliably and also reveal if any of the assessment components need to be modified.

Summary

In this chapter we have looked at reflection as a learning tool and means of enabling lifelong learning through experience, and stressed the need to introduce this early in a learner's education. Clarity and alignment of learning and assessment is needed when we are including reflection in assessment of a programme, particularly in high-stakes' assessments. Of vital importance is the need to define clear aims, SMART learning outcomes, valid, reliable assessments, good feedback and well-trained assessors.

Part IV

Developing as a Reflective Practitioner

11

The Role of Reflection in Developing Professional Identity

> All health professionals go through many processes and encounters on their journey to 'becoming' a professional. Reflection on situations and feelings is a central component of this journey, which may last many years, even a lifetime. This chapter examines how reflective practice can both develop and challenge professional identity formation.

The highest purpose of education is to provide learners with the enabling conditions for self-transformation to newly developed ways of thinking and interacting with others (Goldie, 2012). A career in medicine demands a commitment to lifelong learning and thus requires a continual process of transformation. In medical school, and in the early years of postgraduate training, the transformation is from doing the work of a doctor to becoming one (Jarvis-Selinger, Pratt and Regehr, 2012). Professional identity formation (PIF) is a process influenced directly and indirectly by a great many factors; but it is the reflective process, formal and informal, organized and spontaneous, that facilitates the change and development needed to transform from learner to practitioner.

While reflective practice is vital in PIF, it can challenge an unstable and developing professional (and sometimes personal) identity. In 2015, the UK General Medical Council issued additional guidance around 'Good Medical Practice' entitled 'Openness and honesty when things go wrong: The professional duty of candour' (GMC, 2015). Both doctors and patients might feel concerned at the idea that it should be necessary to provide guidance on something as basic as being open and apologizing for mistakes. Litigation pressure in the clinical environment accounts for a degree of professional self-protection, but a closer look at why doctors struggle with openness and subsequent critical examination of their mistakes raises interesting questions about reflective practice and professional identity.

Developing Reflective Practice: A guide for medical students, doctors and teachers, First Edition.
Andrew Grant, Judy McKimm and Fiona Murphy.
© 2017 John Wiley & Sons Ltd. Published 2017 by John Wiley & Sons Ltd.

A doctor's professional identity begins its development very early, often before entry to medical school (Horsburgh *et al.*, 2006). The title and status of doctor brings with it respect, responsibility and expectations that must be met at each stage of a career; this might reasonably result in the display of an outer confidence that does not necessarily reflect inner feelings. This identity reaches far beyond the workplace: being a doctor carries with it expectations from family, in local communities and among friendship circles. As a result, professional and personal identities are, for doctors, deeply connected (Goldie, 2012). The most effective and productive reflection on personal performance must be honest, critical and at times uncomfortable. In a profession where presenting a confident and competent face is expected at all stages of training, this kind of scrutiny has the potential to be threatening.

How Does Reflective Practice Form Professional Identity?

The explicit teaching of professionalism in medical education in recent decades has evolved to include behaviour, ethics, communication and personal development. This has prompted a dedicated focus in the literature on the principles that underpin PIF for medical students and doctors, these principles including those of professional values and morals as well as professional aspiration and reflection (Holden *et al.*, 2012; Rabow *et al.*, 2010). In functioning as the cornerstone of PIF, reflective practice is also essential in enabling students and doctors to weather the storms of day-to-day clinical life (Mavor *et al.*, 2014). Engaged and regular reflective practice improves resilience, strengthens connections with colleagues and peers and enables individuals to develop techniques for negotiating tricky or potentially disturbing situations (Mavor *et al.*, 2014).

The shift from *doing* to *being* parallels the coming together of an outer and an inner life with regard to professional identity. Leach describes medical professionalism as depending 'heavily on the quality of a physician's inner life' (Leach, 2008, p. 515) and describes the need to embrace a new way of being in order for PIF to occur. Reflection gives the practitioner the opportunity to identify and scrutinize the lived experience and ultimately reconcile the gaps between outer and inner lives. From an ontological perspective, reflection helps people to consider abstract concepts and feelings, to identify what is 'real' for them, what they are going to absorb or reject as part of their professional identity and how this will impact on their practice.

Reflective practice when carried out purposefully and meaningfully results in a more complete practitioner whose professional practice, personal goals and sense of being are synergistic. However, it is not necessarily an intuitive process and is taught (or guided) in various forms during medical training; it is a necessary part of any learning cycle (Pratt, Rockmann and Kaufmann, 2006)

Scenario 11.1 Becoming and being a doctor

Alya decided to spend a year out of training working in Nigeria on a project aimed at strengthening maternal health services in a rural community, prior to applying for obstetrics and gynaecology specialist training in the UK. She is part of a midwife-led team working with local practitioners and village women. After witnessing a number of what she feels should have been preventable child and maternal deaths, she is questioning not only whether she has the will to stay in Africa, but also whether she actually has the emotional capacity to be a doctor anywhere. Telling Carla, their experienced Spanish midwife team leader, about how she feels, she is very surprised when Carla suggests her view on what being a doctor means in reality might be wrong. Carla said that their work here is to work together to improve women's health over the long term, in the meantime they have to support the women and families in the best way they can and that's all they can do. They can't change the world, but they are doing some good. Thinking about this afterwards, she realizes that before she came to Nigeria one of her fundamental reasons for being a doctor was to make people better and she feels she's failed when she can't. She's realised that this just isn't possible, and she needs to take a longer-term perspective of what improving health means and continue to give the best care she can in the circumstances. Carla's wise words have made her really reflect and rethink why she wants to be a doctor and what sort of doctor she wants to be. It'll still be difficult, but she needs to persevere, dig deep and focus on the positive, long-term outcomes for the community.

---

and absolutely fundamental to the process of 'construction, deconstruction and reinterpretation' that is identity formation (Wald, 2015). Intuitive and formalized reflection processes have different yet equally valuable roles. Those who reflect more intuitively should find that formalized, structured reflection consolidates their thinking; those who find active reflection challenging are likely to benefit from a formalized process.

Reflection and critical feedback (formal and informal) play an essential part in forming a secure identity. In this way, reflection as part of day-to-day practice may foster a culture of increased openness in medicine, starting in medical school. Reflective practice also encourages collective notions of success: when positive as well as negative outcomes are considered, the vital role of less prominent team players is recognized and valued differently.

How Can Reflection Be Challenging to Professional Identity?

Gaining entry to medical school requires focus, dedication and a degree of self-promotion. During the undergraduate years the competitive environment encourages students to stand out, to wear an outer confidence and emphasize their strengths and achievements; this culture, which is established early in medical school, continues in the postgraduate training environment. The risk is that this breeds a workforce of 'lone healers' (Lee, 2010) who are poor at forming and working in genuine teams and who think in terms of personal success and failure ahead of team achievements (Mannion, McKimm and O'Sullivan, 2015). For those who lack confidence in their clinical abilities or who fear that isolated failures will give an impression of individual poor performance, any scrutiny of areas that need development might be very uncomfortable. Professional and personal identity in doctors are closely connected, and so the consequences of professional criticism can be far reaching and result in significant personal distress. In more severe cases, people will feel they will be 'found out' or exposed as frauds or imposters, and 'imposter phenomenon' has been found to exist in many professional groups, including doctors and other health professionals (Parkman, 2016). Pressure to perform well (and to appear to perform well) comes from the expectations of professional colleagues but also from patients. In the 2015 Ipsos Mori poll (Ipsos Mori, 2015), doctors retained the position of the nation's most trustworthy professionals. Although patients see a fully formed doctor in every individual they meet who has made it through medical school, for the doctor in training this identity formation is a gradual process that may extend into postgraduate training and beyond, especially when doctors take on new roles or clinical tasks. As vulnerabilities in this developing professional identity are exposed, then individuals may customize by 'patching and splinting' their forming identities with previous ones (Pratt, Rockmann and Kaufmann, 2006). The pressure experienced by medical students and doctors who are attempting to develop an inner identity (that is vulnerable and not yet formed) while projecting an outer professionalism that meets expectations may mean they may be less able to tolerate the scrutiny of formalized reflection, in the form of written reflection or exposing professional conversations. This perceived threat may go some way towards explaining why reflection may prove challenging in some environments, particularly when it is formalized, contributes to assessment or is written down and reviewed by others. It is certainly true that some welcome the reflective process more than others. Self theories may help us to understand how doctors as a group are likely to respond to scrutiny and criticism of performance and attitude, and how this affects attitudes toward reflective practice.

Self Theories, PIF and Reflective Practice

Implicit theories of the self provide a model that can help us to understand how doctors manage challenges to their professional identity and abilities. Implicit theories of the self are domain specific and identify two distinct groups

(Molden and Dweck, 2006). 'Entity' theorists have a fixed, inflexible view of their identity, whereas 'incremental' theorists have a changeable, developmental view of themselves. These self theories may be true across all domains (for example work life, home life, intellectual ability), or differ for the individual in different environments. If professional and personal identity are indeed closely linked in doctors, individuals' theories about their identity are likely to be consistent across domains. Entity theorists, who do not adopt a developmental approach to their identity, will be de-stabilized by direct challenges to the core beliefs they have about themselves. Medical students who hold entity theories will be devastated by disappointing examination results at medical school; incremental theorists will act quickly to identify their weaknesses, and learn and adapt the techniques of those who achieved well.

In the workplace, a doctor who holds entity theories of self will be deeply and personally challenged by criticism of practice generated by even minor oversights or mistakes. Formalized reflection in this context can be very exposing. Those who hold incremental theories are more likely to be natural and constructive reflectors: it is their first reaction to a challenge or disappointment; a formalization of this process will therefore be much less problematic.

A medical career, although rewarding and potentially lucrative, requires highly structured and lengthy training that can feel rigid. The seeds of professional identity are planted at a young age for the majority (Horsburgh *et al.*, 2006). Most new doctors face the immense responsibility of working on a hospital ward in their mid-20s. Many people at this time of life are at a stage of personal discovery and identity formation, while in their professional lives they are often expected to present the face and emotional responses of a fully formed practitioner. Reflection, both formal and informal, is an essential part

---

Scenario 11.2 Coping with failure

Ben has reached the end of his third year at medical school and has failed his written exams. This is the first exam that he has ever failed, having always been top of his class at school. Ben is popular, confident and outspoken and until now he has maintained a very respectable ranking in his year group. He is the first of his family to go to university and his parents are deeply proud of his achievements, his relatives have taken to calling him 'Doctor Ben' and occasionally call him for advice. The only person he has told about the exams is his girlfriend Ellie, who is a medical student in the year below, he has told her not to tell anyone else as he feels ashamed of his results. Ellie offers to sit down with Ben to go through what might have gone wrong, Ben refuses, explaining that she probably wouldn't be able to help him with third year exams as she hasn't reached that level herself yet. Ben privately plans to get through retakes, keeping it all as quiet as possible.

of the development of professional competence and identity. Admissions and assessment culture at medical school encourages competition and ranking and re-enforces the idea that students hold a well-defined position in relation to their peers that is based on their academic abilities. Although reflective practice may be actively taught and encouraged in medical school curricula, the process and results of effective, purposive reflection (focussed on growth, development and change) are not valued and rewarded in the same way as academic attainment.

Scenario 11.3 Asking for help

Grace is one of three FY1 doctors working on a busy respiratory ward in a large district general hospital and is concerned that some of her basic skills are not up to standard. She feels uncertain when assessing acutely unwell patients and about making the less straightforward prescribing decisions, however her fellow FY1s appear very confident and talk a great deal about their daily achievements. She suspects that there is a certain amount of exaggeration involved but her senior colleagues appear to be impressed by them. Grace is dreading a meeting with her educational supervisor to discuss her progress, she would like to ask for support but is terrified of appearing incompetent relative to her peers.

How Can Guided Reflection Be Challenging Without Being Threatening?

Informal guided reflection (which may be spontaneous or organized, in a group setting or one-to-one meeting), by the very fact that it is not recorded or written down, may leave the individual feeling freer to explore challenging ideas. Group settings promote the opportunity for shared experience and understanding of complex scenarios by hearing from different perspectives and opinions. Group reflection is more likely to happen organically, ideas are teased out and multiple perspectives are brought to the table. Communities of practice theory describes groups of people engaging in collective learning in order to achieve common goals (Wenger-Trayner and Wenger-Trayner, 2015); this plays out in formal and informal environments within medicine. This seems to come naturally within many medical communities as learners move along the 'inbound trajectory' to becoming expert, credible members of the medical community. The multiple informal opportunities, such as junior doctors gathering in the mess regularly to discuss how they are managing the day-to-day challenges of ward life, allow for reflection in a much more fluid way. Group problem solving, sharing and reflection of this kind may also serve to model effective, active and routinized reflection to those who find the practice more challenging. It is the more formalized reflective practice, which involves writing or identifying one's own learning needs to a senior, that usually presents a greater challenge. It is understandably difficult to closely examine weaknesses in a professional culture where self-promotion and presenting outer confidence is the norm. While informal and group reflection is extremely valuable, formal and written reflection provides the opportunity for a deeper and more considered understanding of events. Guided reflection in both forms has a significantly formative effect on professional identity. In order for reflective practice to become fully effective, open examination of mistakes and weaknesses without threat must become culturally normal in medicine. The logical place for this shift to start is in medical school, where reflective practice in all elements of learning should be the norm. Doctors and doctors-to-be should not only be ethically sound, honest and competent but have the skills of self-examination that help to build rather than threaten professional identity.

Summary

For PIF to occur, the necessary ingredients are 'include experiential and reflective processes, guided reflection, formative feedback, use of personal narratives… role models and candid discussion within a safe community of learners' (Wald, 2015, p. 2). Reflective practice can, at the same time, be empowering and threatening in an environment where identity is in the process of development. A professional culture that supports and encourages the examination of weaknesses and exposure of vulnerability (as well as the celebration of success) is vital if guided reflective practice is to have a genuine impact on thinking, doing and being. Engaged and challenging reflection gradually brings together the outer fully fledged professional and the inner 'doctor-under-construction', the ultimate goal being to nurture a confident and competent practitioner who has the skills to adapt, learn and develop as a professional from the point of entry to medical school to the day of retirement.

Reflection, Revalidation and Appraisal

This chapter considers the role of reflection in training, lifelong learning and continuing professional development, with a particular focus on the appraisal and revalidation processes. Whilst considering how best to compile a body of satisfactory evidence for revalidation and how to structure the appraisal to incorporate reflection, the chapter also looks more deeply into the underpinning processes and how these can aid or inhibit reflection.

We will apply much of the theoretical and practical information described in previous chapters to the business of using reflection in order to keep up to date in the constantly changing world of medicine and other healthcare professions, while at the same time demonstrating that this reflective-learning activity has taken place.

Adult Learning – Andragogy

Many writers, in particular Malcolm Knowles, have identified that children and adults learn differently. Knowles, Holton and Swanson (2005) cite the work of another American educator, Eduard C. Lindemann (Lindemann, 1926), who believed that for adult learners the curriculum should be built around the interests of the learner. Lindemann's key assumptions about adult learners are shown in Box 12.1.

Although the concepts underpinning andragogy are relevant throughout this book, they are particularly relevant when considering reflective learning in continuing professional development. In *The Adult Learner*, Knowles and colleagues build on earlier work and note six features that distinguish adult

Developing Reflective Practice: A guide for medical students, doctors and teachers, First Edition.
Andrew Grant, Judy McKimm and Fiona Murphy.

> **Box 12.1 Lindemann's five key assumptions about adult learning (cited by Knowles, Holton and Swanson, 2005)**
>
> 1) Adults are motivated to learn as they experience needs and interests that learning will satisfy.
> 2) Adults' orientation to learning is life centred.
> 3) Experience is the richest source for adults' learning.
> 4) Adults have a deep need to be self-directing.
> 5) Individual differences among people increase with age.

learning from pedagogy (educating children), which we will consider in relation to reflective practice as part of continuing professional development:

1) the need to know;
2) the learners' self-concept;
3) the role of the learners' experiences;
4) readiness to learn;
5) orientations to learning;
6) motivation.

1. The Need to Know

A busy practitioner is unlikely to invest time and effort in learning something when they do not or cannot see *the need to know*. Although learners of all ages are likely to do better if they can see that they are learning something of some relevance and/or importance to them, adults, who are more used to being autonomous and making decisions about their own lives, are particularly unlikely to engage in learning something they do not see as relevant. Learning linked directly to the workplace, identified through personal interest, a need to better understand specific patients' conditions or obtained through solicited feedback is likely to be seen as more relevant.

2. The Learners' Self-Concept

Adults being used to deciding for themselves what they do and don't do (and do and don't learn) is an important expression of *the learners' self-concept*. For many adult learners, having to go back into a classroom and learn whatever is presented to them by a teacher is likely to feel like being forced back to their childhood or adolescence. This might also lead to their behaviour reverting to that stage in their development. So being able to access online or other forms of open access learning linked to their *need to know* might help busy adult learners retain their self-concept and agency.

3. The Role of the Learners' Experiences

We talked about experiential learning as a model for learning using reflection in Chapter 3. For an adult using reflection as a basis for continued professional development, the *role of the learners' experiences* is key. We are used to the curriculum being determined by the people who design the course and set the assessments in school and university. However, for the adult learner wanting to undertake tailor-made learning relevant to their daily practice, it is their personal experiences that form the 'curriculum' (the course of study). Moreover, it is reflection that helps them to unpack the learning content from these experiences and turn them into learning objectives (what they want or need to learn), learning plans (the methods and timing of learning) and finally new knowledge or understanding that they can apply in their practice.

4. Readiness to Learn

Interlinked with the role of learners' experiences is their *readiness to learn*. This can arise from a number of triggers: it may be a critical event, but it equally may be as simple as wanting to keep up to date to do the best for your patients. We give an example of readiness to learn in conjunction with *Orientations to learning* and *Motivation*; see Scenario 12.1.

5. Orientations to Learning

The way in which students come across learning opportunities will make a significant difference to whether or not they connect with students' *orientation to learning*. Because their curriculum is set by their experience, adult learners are looking for learning that can improve their proficiency in their daily life, including their working life.

6. Motivation

All adults desire to continue growing and developing and it is this sense of *motivation* from within them that is the force most likely to drive their learning. Where learners are not engaging in learning that will help them grow and

Scenario 12.1

Katy, a GP, is about to take on a new role in the practice, looking after patients newly diagnosed with diabetes. She quickly realizes that her ability to look after these patients is held back by her lack of knowledge of the modes of action of the numerous new antidiabetic drugs released onto the market. Her 'learning objectives' are therefore to learn about these drugs to identify which might be the most appropriate for the different groups of patients under her care. She is now ready to learn about them, and has both the internal and external motivation to do so. Six months previously, when caring for these patients was the responsibility of another doctor in the practice, she was less ready. This is an important point. What is learned and how it is learned is determined by the learner, by their experience, by what is going on in their lives.

Katy is a busy GP with family commitments, and she tends to do her reading and updating in the evenings once the children are in bed. Doing some online searching and asking colleagues about suitable ways to acquire this new knowledge, although numerous scientific articles exist about the mechanisms of different drugs and there are short courses run by the local Trust, she is most attracted to a recently developed online learning module ('the curriculum') reviewed in the BMJ entitled 'A staged approach to prescribing in diabetes', which has an inbuilt self-testing feature. This forms the basis of her 'learning plan'; she can do this module over the next couple of weeks, which fits well with work and home commitments. She feels that she has confidence in the content of the module, and once she has completed the learning and assessment she will be much more competent to look after these patients. The way she chooses to learn reflects both her orientation to learning and self-concept as a learner and health professional.

develop this may be due not to lack of intrinsic motivation but to barriers such as their belief in their own ability to address their learning needs or to circumstantial obstacles such as lack of time or opportunity.

Maximizing Learning Return on Effort

As we have discussed in previous chapters, it is important to recognize that, as a medical or healthcare practitioner, you will be expected to invest a significant amount of time in reflective-learning activities that keep you up to date with the constant changes in knowledge and practices of your profession. You will always be expected to demonstrate that this activity has taken place. Through reflection, you will need to demonstrate that you are thinking about your practice, your interactions with patients and their families and how fit your knowledge and training makes you for the job that you do. From these, you will identify things you need to know or change and provide examples of these as evidence of *reflection for action*.

A Curriculum Based on Your Experience

In this section we will look at how to develop a curriculum tailored to your own needs based on your own experience. The questions in Boxes 12.2 and 12.3 have been designed to help you to reflect critically on your own experience and identify your learning needs. The list is not meant to be exhaustive and you might want to develop alternative questions that better fit your own circumstances and learning needs.

Using critical questions such as these will help you to ensure that the time and energy you expend on reflecting on your practice and keeping up to date

---

Box 12.2 Reflection in relation to interactions with individual patients

- Did that patient leave satisfied with the encounter?
  - If they did, what did you do to make that happen? On reflection is there anything you might have done differently?
  - If they did not, what could I learn to help in future patient encounters?

- Was my core knowledge[1] adequate to deal with that patient's problem?
  - If not what deficits were brought to light?
  - How do you plan to address them?

- Did I have the necessary communication and procedural skills to deal with that patient and their concerns?
  - If not what are the gaps? How do you plan to address them?

- Was there any aspect of that patient encounter you found difficult? (for example was there anything you found upsetting or challenging?)
  - Why was this so?

- What was it about this encounter that was similar to and different from others?

[1] Whilst most practitioners will need and expect to look up certain information on a routine basis there is some knowledge (that we call 'core') that all practitioners in a particular specialty might be expected to be able to recall and apply from memory. What constitutes core knowledge is determined by the specialty, the level of seniority and, to some extent, by each individual practitioner.

Box 12.3 Reflection on practice over time

- What kind of patient encounters make you feel that you are doing a worthwhile job?
  - Do you know what it is about these patients that make you feel like this? Does this represent an area of special interest for you?
- What kind of patients make your heart sink?
  - Can you be specific why they have this effect on you?
  - Can you do any special training or change the way you or your service works to minimize this effect?
- Have you received any complaints from patients?
  - How did that make you feel?
  - How did you deal with the complaint?
  - Were you able to learn from the process?
- Are there areas of your work that don't directly involve patient contact (e.g. education, clinical governance, management, leadership)? Rate how much you enjoy these aspects of your work on a scale of 1 to 10 where 1 = dislike them intensely and 10 = enjoy very much.
  - If you have scored these activities highly what is it about them that you enjoy?
  - If you have given these activities a low score what is it about them that you dislike? Can you undergo any training that will help with this? Are there areas of your work you can drop or change?
- What areas of the service you help provide for your patients makes you proud?
- What areas of the service you help provide do you wish would change in some way?
  - How can you start to make these changes happen?

---

will give you the best possible return on the time invested. This may bring about a conflict where you feel that you just don't have enough time to spend on your reflective learning, and sometimes that will probably be true. You may also feel that all you need to do is to satisfy the person who is evaluating your portfolio for appraisal and determining whether you have in fact undergone sufficient [reflective] learning activity. If you ask a practitioner how they would like their knowledge and skills relating to their profession to be, almost everyone would say that they wanted to have a good, appropriate level of knowledge for the job that they were doing. However, if you ask a practitioner who has to complete their portfolio for appraisal (particularly if they have left it to that last minute and it has to be submitted online by 0900 the following day) what their immediate goal is, they may well say that it is producing a document that will satisfy their appraiser or assessor. These two outcomes may be very different indeed.

So what can we do to ensure the best possible outcome from these learning activities? We suggest that the first thing is to recognize

- the kind of practitioner that we wish to be;
- the kind of learning outcomes that we want to get from continuing professional development activities;
- that *intrinsically motivated learning relating to personal experience* is different from any other forms of learning.

In Activity 12.1, we suggest how you might use a previous experience of an episode of intrinsically motivated, self-directed learning to identify some aspects of how you learn, what you learn, how you feel about it and how you apply this learning to action.

The purpose of this exercise is to help you to recognize that you already have an inbuilt capacity for learning from experience (as described in adult-learning theory above) and that you are able to do this in a way that is associated with positive affect and a positive sense of self-efficacy.

Activity 12.1 Learning from learning

Think about an episode of learning, formal or informal, when you were able to change your understanding of the subject in relation to a particular instance or a particular patient: in other words, an 'experience'.

- What was it that made you realize that learning had taken place?
- How did learning in that way make you feel?
- Is this learning that you think you have and/or you will retain over time?
- What can you learn from this for future learning experiences?

Learning that is Intrinsically Rewarding

If your time spent in continuous professional development is related to activities you enjoy and get satisfaction from, the activity itself will be the reward. Intrinsically motivated learning is associated with a sense of being a better person in some way (perhaps with better knowledge and therefore being better able to do the job), what the humanistic psychologists would call 'self-actualisation'. This is when you maximize your potential and do the best that you are capable of. Maslow (1987) (best known for his 'hierarchy of needs') suggests that self-actualized people have the following characteristics:

- they embrace and are attracted by the unknown, the ambiguous and the mysterious – they have a thirst to find out 'why?';

- they accept themselves with human flaws, yet seek to change the things that they can such as deficits and bad habits;
- they enjoy experiences and activities intrinsically, not just as a means to an end;
- they are motivated by personal growth, not just the satisfaction of physical and psychological needs;
- they are humble, know they're imperfect and are willing to learn from anyone or anything.

The drive towards self-actualization is seen as a basic human motivator, and we know too that when learners feel good about themselves this is associated with sustained, integrated learning. A practitioner who is undergoing learning like this, based on episodes in their practice on a regular basis, will be self-motivated, will be able to keep up to date and will have a very positive sense of their own knowledge and ability to learn. They will also take a lead on their own learning and knowledge development. This is very different from the didactic, traditional approach to education, in which what is learned is determined by the teacher rather than the individual learner.

Keeping a Record for CPD, Appraisal and Revalidation

Although reflective learning is rewarding in itself, and the best possible way to find out is to experience it for yourself, if you are a practitioner you will be expected to produce evidence of your reflective learning, and either to submit it in electronic or written form to your appraiser or to present your reflective learning orally. This collection of evidence is often referred to as a portfolio for appraisal. And as we have discussed in previous chapters, this is often asked for in the form of a series of learning encounters, recorded using various reflective-learning templates in a web-based format. The purpose of these templates is to help you, the learner, work through the stages of whichever reflective-learning cycle you choose to demonstrate that a full cycle of reflective learning has taken place. It is also designed to help you to maximize your reflective-learning potential. Chapter 4 describes commonly used frameworks for reflection including those of Borton (1970), Kolb (1984), Gibbs (1988) and Rolfe, Jasper and Freshwater (2011).

You will need to find a way of meeting the formal written requirements of appraisal that enhance rather than detract from your reflective-learning activity. We have mentioned before that learners often refer to reflective learning as a 'tick-box activity'. If you find yourself thinking about reflection like this, it is worth asking yourself whether there is anything you can do differently to make this a more meaningful reflective-learning activity, not one simply driven by the requirements of a course or the regulator. It will be helpful for your appraiser or assessor if you can set out as clearly as possible:

- what you set out to do in a particular episode of reflective learning;
- what you got out of it
  - what you learned,
  - how you think your understanding has changed;
- how you think your practice might change in the future.

Demonstrating Learning and Development over Time

As we discussed in Chapter 10, if you are constructing a portfolio over a period of time, then it is very important to take the opportunity to explain how your understanding or development has developed in a particular area over time. It is also important to write entries in your portfolio and to add other material that helps to express what you are trying to say, that is particularly relevant to you. A portfolio and a reflective-learning entry in it should be highly personal, and should enable you to express things in a way that you feel comfortable with. If the particular headings of the template do not fit the work you are trying to do then say so and possibly adapt them for your needs.

In terms of metacognition (thinking about thinking), a portfolio for appraisal, written over a period of time with references forward and back showing how your understanding has changed over time and the things that have changed it, should show significant evidence of metacognitive activity. You are not simply reproducing knowledge, but taking charge of what knowledge you acquire, how you acquire it and how it is applied to your own practice and professional development.

Box 12.4 Extract from professional development portfolio

There are two main ways in which I feel I have changed over the course of the programme. Firstly, I have learnt the importance of self-reflection and how to use it as a tool for my own development. At the start of the programme I was sceptical about the value of reflective practice, having been introduced to it vaguely through passing activities in my undergraduate education and within my online e-portfolio as a doctor in training. The program, through its many interactive sessions, has taught me that effective self-reflection requires realisation of our limitations and weaknesses first before we can bring about a change. In particular, I found the model by Proctor on moving from novice to expert helpful by thinking about your own unconscious incompetence and conscious incompetence (Proctor 2001). Reflection requires a dialogic process which can occur internally or externally and I have begun to more consciously try to seek out opportunities to engage in constructive feedback to this end. Ultimately, I have come to understand the reflective practice is an iterative cycle and takes time. It is not switched on and off whenever you need to fill in a free text box as part of an imposed exercise. Over time, mindfulness either by learning theory or observing the habits of others, can trigger a realisation within yourself and bring about a change as described in Kolb's Learning Cycle (Kolb 1976). Better understanding of the way we learn and how self-reflection fits in to self development has meant that I have adopted it as a technique for maturing in both my personal and professional life.

(Written by doctor in training on leadership programme.)

Summary

This chapter has focussed on reflection in the context of the qualified, experienced practitioner who is required to produce a portfolio for revalidation and/or appraisal. However, despite the external demands on health practitioners to engage in reflective activities, we have also shown that purposeful, conscious reflection forms a key part of enjoyable, satisfying and meaningful learning for its own sake.

References and Resources

References

Alsop, A. and Ryan, S. (1996) *Making the Most of Fieldwork Education*,cited in McClure, P. *Reflection on Practice*. Making Practice Based Learning Work, http://cw.routledge.com/textbooks/9780415537902/data/learning/8_Reflection%20in%20Practice.pdf (accessed 2 January 2017).

Anderson, L.W., Krathwohl, D.R. and Bloom, B.S. (2001) *A Taxonomy for Learning, Teaching, and Assessing: A Revision of Bloom's Taxonomy of Educational Objectives*, Allyn & Bacon.

Argyris, C., Putnam, R. and Smith, D.M. (1985) *Action Science: Concepts, Methods and Skills for Research and Intervention*, Jossey Bass, San Francisco.

Ausubel, D.P. (2000) *The Acquisition and Retention of Knowledge*, Kluwer Academic Publishers, Dordrecht, The Netherlands.

Bandura, A. (1997) *Self-Efficacy: The Exercise of Control*, W.H. Freeman, New York.

Bassot, B. (2012) *The Reflective Diary. Enhancing Professional Development*, Matador.

Bergold, J. and Thomas, S. (2012) Participatory research methods: a methodological approach in motion. *Forum: Qualitative Social Research*, **13** (1), Art. 30.

Biggs, J. and Tang, A. (2011) *Learning to Teach in Higher Education: What the Student Does*, 4th edn, Open University Press, Maidenhead, UK.

Borton, T. (1970) *Reach, Touch and Teach*, Hutchinson, London.

Boud, D., Keogh, R. and Walker, D. (1985) Promoting reflection in learning: A model, in *Reflection: Turning Experience into Learning* (eds D. Boud, R. Keogh and D. Walker), Kogan Page, London, pp. 18–40.

Bourner, T. (2003) Assessing reflective learning. *Education + Training*, **45**, 267.

Bowman, M. and Addyman, B. (2014) Academic reflective writing: A study to examine its usefulness. *British Journal of Nursing*, **23** (6), 304–309.

Brady, D.W., Corbie-Smith, G. and Branch, W.T. Jr (2002) "What's important to you?": The use of narratives to promote self-reflection and to understand the experiences of medical residents. *Annals of Internal Medicine*, **137**, 220–223,cited in Branch, W.T. (2005) Use of critical incident reports in medical education:

Developing Reflective Practice: A guide for medical students, doctors and teachers, First Edition.
Andrew Grant, Judy McKimm and Fiona Murphy.
© 2017 John Wiley & Sons Ltd. Published 2017 by John Wiley & Sons Ltd.

A perspective. *Journal of General Internal Medicine*, **20** (11), 1063–1067, http://www.ncbi.nlm.nih.gov/pmc/articles/PMC1490252/ (accessed 3 January 2017).

Bringle, R.G. and Hatcher, J.A. (1999) Reflection in service learning: Making meaning of experience. *Educational Horizons, Summer*, 179–185,cited in Sloan, D. and Hartsfield, T.S. *Section 3. Reflection Activities*, http://www.aacc.nche.edu/Resources/aaccprograms/horizons/Documents/reflection_3.pdf (accessed 3 January 2017).

Brockbank, A. and McGill, I. (2009) *Facilitating Reflective Learning in Higher Education*, 2nd edn, Open University Press.

Brookfield, S. (1987) *Developing Critical Thinkers*, Open University Press, Milton Keynes, UK.

Brookfield, S. (1998) Critically reflective practice. *Journal of Continuing Education in the Health Professions*, **18**, 197–205.

Bruner, J. (1996) *The Culture of Education*, Harvard University Press, Cambridge, MA.

Bruning, R., Schraw, G. and Norby, M. (2011) *Cognitive Psychology and Instruction*, 5th edn, Pearson Education Inc., Boston, MA.

Carr, W. and Kemmis, S. (1986) *Becoming Critical: Education, Knowledge and Action Research*, Routledge, London.

COBE (2005) *Action Research: A Guide for Associate Lecturers*, Open University.

Comer, M. (2016) Rethinking reflection-in-action: What did Schön really mean? *Nurse Education Today*, **36**, 4–6.

Cooperrider, D. and Whitney, D.D. (2005) *Appreciative Inquiry: A Positive Revolution in Change*, Berrett-Koehler Publishers.

Criticos, C. (1993) Experiential learning and social transformation for a post-apartheid learning future, in *Using Experience for Learning* (ed. D. Boud, R. Cohen and D. Walker), Society for Research into Higher Education and Open University Press, pp. 157–168.

Cross, T.A. and Angelo, K.P. (1993) *Classroom Assessment Techniques: A Handbook for College Teachers*, Jossey-Bass Publishers, San Francisco.

de Bono, E. (1985) *Six Thinking Hats*. Penguin Publishers.

De Souza, B. and Viney, R. (2014) Coaching and mentoring skills: necessities for today's doctors. *BMJ Careers*, http://careers.bmj.com/careers/advice/view-article.html?id=20018242 (accessed 3 January 2017).

Delany, C. and Golding, C. (2014) Teaching clinical reasoning by making thinking visible: An action research project with allied health clinical educators. *BMC Medical Education*, **14**, 20, http://bmcmededuc.biomedcentral.com/articles/10.1186/1472-6920-14-20 (accessed 3 January 2017).

Dewey, J. (1910) *How We Think*, D.C. Heath, Boston, MA.

Doctors' Defence Service UK (2016) *Reflective Writing in GMC Cases – Showing Insight*, https://doctorsdefenceservice.com/showing-insight-in-reflective-writing-in-gmc-cases/ (accessed 3 August 2016).

Downey, M. (2003) *Effective Coaching*, 3rd edn, Thomson Texere.

Driscoll, J. (2007) *Practising Clinical Supervision: A Reflective Approach for Healthcare Professionals*, 2nd edn, Bailliere Tindall Elsevier, Edinburgh.

Finlay, L. (2008) *Reflecting on 'Reflective Practice'*, PBPL Paper 52, The Open University.

Flanagan, J.C. (1954) The critical incident technique. *Psychological Bulletin*, **51** (4), https://www.apa.org/pubs/databases/psycinfo/cit-article.pdf (accessed 3 January 2017).

Freire, P. (1970) *Pedagogy of the Oppressed*, Herder and Herder, New York.

Freire, P. (1996) *Pedagogy of the Oppressed*, Penguin Books, London.

General Medical Council (GMC) (2009) *Tomorrows Doctors*, GMC, London.

General Medical Council (GMC) (2013) *Doctors' Use of Social Media*, http://www.gmc-uk.org/guidance/ethical_guidance/21186.asp (accessed 3 January 2017).

General Medical Council (GMC) (2014) *The Meaning of Fitness to Practise*, http://www.gmc-uk.org/the_meaning_of_fitness_to_practise.pdf_25416562.pdf (accessed 3 August 2016).

General Medical Council (GMC) (2015) Openness and honesty when things go wrong: The professional duty of candour, in *Good Medical Practice, GMC*, http://www.gmc-uk.org/guidance/ethical_guidance/27233.asp (accessed 26 April 2016).

generationOn (2011) *Service Learning Reflection Activities by Type and Length*, http://www.generationon.org/files/flat-page/files/checklist_of_reflection_activities.pdf (accessed 3 January 2017).

Gibbs, G. (1988) *Learning by Doing: A Guide to Teaching and Learning*, Oxford Centre for Staff and Learning Development, Oxford. http://www2.glos.ac.uk/gdn/gibbs/index.htm (accessed 3 January 2017).

Giddens, A. (1991) *Modernity and Self-Identity*, Stanford University Press, Stanford, CA.

Gijselaers, W. (1995) Perspectives on problem-based learning, in *Educational Innovation in Economics and Business Administration: The Case of Problem-Based Learning* (eds W. Gijselaers, D. Tempelaar, P. Keizer *et al.*), Kluwer, Dordrecht, The Netherlands, pp. 39–52.

Goldie, J. (2012) The formation of professional identity in medical students: Considerations for educators. *Medical Teacher*, **34** (9), e641–e648.

Goldsmith, S. (1995) *Journal Reflection: A Resource Guide for Community Service Leaders and Educators Engaged in Service Learning*, American Alliance for Rights and Responsibilities, Washington, DC.

Grant, A. (2013) *Reflection and Medical Students' Learning. An In-Depth Study Combining Qualitative and Quantitative Methods*. Lambert Academic Publishing

Grant, A., Berlin, A. and Freeman, G.K. (2003) The impact of a student learning journal: An evaluation using the nominal group technique. *Medical Teacher*, **25**, 335–340.

Grant, A., Kinnersley, P., Metcalff, E. *et al.* (2006) Students' views of reflective learning techniques: An efficacy study at a UK medical school. *Medical Education*, **40**, 379–388.

Greenhalgh, T., Howick, J. and Maskrey, N. (2014) Evidence based medicine: A movement in crisis? *BMJ* **2014**, 348, g3725.

Greenwood, D.J. and Levin, M. (2007) *Introduction to Action Research*, 2nd edn, Sage, Thousand Oaks, CA.

Heron, J. (1976) A six-category intervention analysis. *British Journal of Guidance and Counselling*, **4** (2), 143–155.

Heron, J. (1986) *Six Category Intervention Analysis*, 2nd edn, Human Potential Research Project, University of Guildford, UK.

Heron, J. (1996) *Co-operative Inquiry: Research into the Human Condition*, Sage, London.

Herr, K. and Anderson, G.L. (2005) *The Action Research Dissertation: A Guide for Students and Faculty*, Sage, Thousand Oaks, CA.

Hodgson, A.K. and Scanlan, J.M. (2013) A concept analysis of mentoring in nursing leadership. *Open Journal of Nursing*, **3**, 389–394. doi: org/10.4236/ojn.2013.35052

Holden, M., Buck, E., Clark, M. *et al.* (2012) Professional Identity Formation in medical education; The convergence of multiple domains. *HEC Forum*, **24**, 245–255.

Horsburgh, M., Perkins, R., Coyle, B. and Degeling, P. (2006) The professional subcultures of students entering medical, nursing and pharmacy programmes. *Journal of Interprofessional Care*, **20** (4), 425–431. doi: 10.1080/13561820600805233

Huang, H.B. (2010) What is good action research?: Why the resurgent interest? *Action Research*, **8**, 93.

INVOLVE (2009) *Research Design Services and Public Involvement*, INVOLVE, Eastleigh, UK.

Ipsos Mori (2015) *Politicians Trusted Less than Estate Agents, Bankers and Journalists*, Ipsos Mori, https://www.ipsos-mori.com/researchpublications/researcharchive/3685/Politicians-are-still-trusted-less-than-estate-agents-journalists-and-bankers.aspx (accessed 3 January 2017).

Jarvis-Selinger, S., Pratt, D.D. and Regehr, G. (2012) Competency is not enough: Integrating identity formation into medical education discourse. *Academic Medicine*, **87**, 1185–1190.

Jasper, M. (2006) *Professional Development, Reflection and Decision-Making*, Blackwell, Oxford.

Jasper, M. (2008) Using reflective journals and diaries to enhance practice and learning, in *Reflective Practice in Nursing*, 4th edn (eds C. Bulman and S. Schutz), Blackwell, Chichester, pp. 163–188.

Jasper, M. (2013) *Beginning Reflective Practice*, Cengage Learning, Andover, UK.

Kehlet, H. (1997) Multimodal approach to control postoperative pathophysiology and rehabilitation. *British Journal of Anaesthesia*, **78**, 606–617.

King, P.M., and Kitchener, K.S. (1994) *Developing Reflective Judgment: Understanding and Promoting Intellectual Growth and Critical Thinking in Adolescents and Adults*, Jossey-Bass, San Francisco.

Knowles, M., Holton, E. and Swanson, R. (2005) *The Adult Learner*, Elsevier, Burlington, MA.

Kolb, D.A. (1984) *Experiential Learning: Experience as a Source of Learning and Development*. Prentice-Hall, Englewood Cliffs, NJ.

Koole, S., Dornan, T., Leen, A. *et al.* (2011) Factors confounding the assessment of reflection: a critical review. *BMC Medical Education*, 11.

Kouzes, J.M. and Posner, B.Z. (2009) The Five Practices of Exemplary Leadership, in *The Jossey-Bass Reader on Educational Leadership*, Jossey-Bass, San Francisco, pp. 63–72.

Krause, S. (1996) Portfolios in teacher education: Effects of instruction on preservice teachers' early comprehension of the portfolio process. *Journal of Teacher Education*, **47**, 130–138.

Lave, J. and Wenger, E. (1991) *Situated Learning: Legitimate Peripheral Participation*, Cambridge University Press, Cambridge.

Leach, D.C. (2008) Medical professionalism and the formation of residents: A journey towards authenticity. *University of St Thomas Law Journal*, **5**, 21–521.

Lee, T.H. (2010) Turning doctors into leaders. *Harvard Business Review*, **88** (4), 50–58.

Lewin, K. (1946). Action research and minority problems. *Journal of Social Issues*, **2** (4), 34–46.

Lindemann, E. (1926) *The Meaning of Adult Learning*, New Republic, New York.

Mahajan, R.P. (2010) Critical incident reporting and learning. *British Journal of Anaesthetics*, **105** (1), 69-75. doi: 10.1093/bja/aeq133

Mannion, H., McKimm, J. and O'Sullivan, H. (2015) Followership, clinical leadership and social identity. *British Journal of Hospital Medicine*, **76** (5), 270–274.

Marton, F., Hounsell, D. and Entwistle, N. (eds) (1997) *The Experience of Learning*, Scottish Academic Press, Edinburgh.

Marton, F. and Säljö, R. (1997) Approaches to learning, in *The Experience of Learning* (eds F. Marton, D. Hounsell and N. Entwistle), Scottish Academic Press, Edinburgh, pp. 39–58.

Maslach, C. (1982) *Burnout: The Cost of Caring*, Prentice Hall.

Maslow, A. (1987) *Motivation and Personality*, Harper and Row.

Mathers, N., Mitchell, C. and Hunn, A. (2012) *A Study to Assess the Impact of Continuing Professional Development (CPD) on Doctors' Performance and Patient/Service Outcomes for the GMC*. University of Sheffield.

Matthews, R. (2014) Additional barriers to clinical supervision for allied health professionals working in regional and remote settings. *Australian Health Review*, **38** (1), 118.

Mavor, K.L., McNeill, K.G., Anderson, K. *et al.* (2014) Beyond prevalence to process: The role of self and identity in medical student well-being. *Medical Education*, **48**, 351–360.

McClure, P. (2005) *Reflection on Practice: Making Practice Based Learning work*, http://cw.routledge.com/textbooks/9780415537902/data/learning/8_Reflection%20in%20Practice.pdf (accessed 3 January 2017).

Mendenhall, T.J. and Doherty, W.J. (2007) Partners in diabetes. Action research in a primary care setting. *Action Research*, **5** (4), 378–406.

MindTools (2016) *Heron's Six Categories of Intervention*, www.mindtools.com/CommSkll/HeronsCategories.htm (accessed 18 July 2016).

Molden, D.C. and Dweck, C.S. (2006) Finding 'meaning' in psychology: A lay theories approach to self-regulation, social perception and social development. *American Psychology*, **61** (3), 192–203.

Moon, J. (1999) *Reflection in Learning and Professional Development*, Kogan Page, London.

Morton-Cooper, A. (2000) *Action Research in Health Care*, Blackwell Science, Oxford.

Newton, P. and Burgess, D. (2008) Exploring types of educational action research: Implications for research validity. *International Journal of Qualitative Methods*, **7** (4), 18–30.

O'Sullivan, G., Hocking, C. and Spence, D. (2014) Action research: Changing history for people living with dementia in New Zealand. *Action Research*, **12** (1), 19–35.

Parkman, A. (2016) The imposter phenomenon in higher education: Incidence and impact. *Journal of Higher Education Theory and Practice*, **16** (1), 51–60.

Perry, S. (2014) *A Kindness*, Poetry Space Ltd.

Perry, W.G. Jr (1970) *Forms of Intellectual and Ethical Development in the College Years: A Scheme*, Holt, Rinehart, and Winston, New York.

Pink, J., Cadbury, N. and Stanton, N. (2008) Enhancing student reflection: The development of an e-portfolio. *Medical Education*, **42**, 1132–1133.

Pratt, M.G., Rockmann, K.W. and Kaufmann, J.B. (2006) Constructing professional identity: The role of work identity learning cycles in the customization of identity among medical residents. *Academy of Management Journal*, **49** (2), 235–262.

Rabow, M.W., Reme, R.N., Parmelee, D.X. and Inui, T.S. (2010) Professional formation: Extending medicine's lineage of service into the next century. *Academic Medicine*, **85**, 310–317.

Reason, P. and Rowan, J. (eds) (1981) *Human Inquiry: A Sourcebook of New Paradigm Research*, John Wiley & Sons, Ltd, Chichester, UK, pp. 395–399.

Reed, E., Cullen, A., Gannon, C. *et al.* (2015) Use of Schwartz Centre Rounds in a UK hospice: Findings from a longitudinal evaluation. *Journal of Interprofessional Care*, **29** (4), 365–366. doi: 10.3109/13561820.2014.983594

Rolfe, G. (2014) Rethinking reflective education: What would Dewey have done? *Nurse Education Today*, **34**, 1179–1183.

Rolfe, G., Jasper, M. and Freshwater, D. (2011) *Critical Reflection in Practice. Generating Knowledge for Care*, 2nd edn, Palgrave Macmillan, Basingstoke, UK.

Sackett, D.L. *et al.* (1996) Evidence based medicine: what it is and what it isn't. *BMJ*, **312**, 71.

Sandars, J. (2008) Reflective learning and the net generation. *Medical Teacher*, **30**, 877.

Schön, D.A. (1983) *The Reflective Practitioner: How Professionals Think in Action*, Temple Smith, London.

Schön, D.A. (1987) *Educating the Reflective Practitioner*, Jossey-Bass, San Francisco.

Schön, D.A. (1992) The crisis of professional knowledge and the pursuit of an epistemology of practice. *Journal of Interprofessional Care*, **6** (1), 49–63.

Surgenor, P. (2011) *Tutor, Demonstrator & Coordinator Development. Reflective Practice*, http://www.ucd.ie/t4cms/Reflective%20Practice.pdf (accessed 3 January 2017).

Taylor, B. (2010) *Reflective Practice for Healthcare Professionals*, 3rd edn, Open University Press, Maidenhead, UK.

Vygotsky, L. (1978) *Mind in Society: The Development of Higher Psychological Processes*, Harvard University Press, Cambridge, MA.

Wald, H.S. (2015) Professional identity (trans)formation: Reflection, relationship, resilience. *Academic Medicine*, **90** (6), 1–6.

Wenger-Trayner, E. and Wenger-Trayner, B. (2015) *Introduction to Communities of Practice: A Brief Overview of the Concept and its Uses*, http://wenger-trayner.com/introduction-to-communities-of-practice/ (accessed 3 January 2017).

Whitmore, J. (2009) *Coaching for Performance*, 4th edn, Nicholas Brealey Publishing, London.

Further Resources

http://qmplus.qmul.ac.uk/mod/book/view.php?id=257889

http://www.nottingham.ac.uk/nmp/sonet/rlos/placs/critical_reflection/models/index.html

http://www.open.edu/openlearn/education/learning-teach-becoming-reflective-practitioner/content-section-6.3

http://www.monash.edu.au/lls/llonline/writing/medicine/reflective/2.1.xml

http://www.ndm.ox.ac.uk/grace-irimu-participatory-action-research-in-clinical-settings http://www.usf.edu/engagement/documents/nwtoolkit.pdf

Index

Index for *Developing Reflective Practice*

Developing Reflective Practice: A guide for medical students, doctors and teachers, First Edition.
Andrew Grant, Judy McKimm and Fiona Murphy.
© 2017 John Wiley & Sons Ltd. Published 2017 by John Wiley & Sons Ltd.